HEMODYNAMIC BASIS OF ATHEROSCLEROSIS

HEMODYNAMIC BASIS OF ATHEROSCLEROSIS

Meyer Texon, M.D.
New York University Medical Center
and
Office of the Chief Medical Examiner
of the City of New York

HEMISPHERE PUBLISHING CORPORATION
Washington New York London

IN COOPERATION WITH

McGRAW-HILL INTERNATIONAL BOOK COMPANY

New York St. Louis San Francisco Auckland Beirut Bogotá
Düsseldorf Johannesburg Lisbon London Lucerne Madrid
Mexico Montreal New Delhi Panama Paris San Juan
São Paulo Singapore Sydney Tokyo Toronto

HEMODYNAMIC BASIS OF ATHEROSCLEROSIS

1 2 3 4 5 6 7 8 9 0 M K M K 7 8 3 2 1 0 9

Library of Congress Cataloging in Publication Data

Texon, Meyer, date.
Hemodynamic basis of atherosclerosis.

Bibliography: p.
Includes index.
1. Atherosclerosis—Etiology. 2. Hemodynamics.
I. Title. [DNLM: 1. Atherosclerosis—Etiology.
2. Hemodynamics. WG550 T355h]
RC692.T49 616.1'36 79-4466
Hemisphere ISBN 0-89116-146-5
McGraw-Hill ISBN 0-07-063765-2

To my wife, Ami
To my son, Stephen
To my daughter, Sylvia

CONTENTS

FOREWORD

Claude Bernard wrote, "We are all fallible when facing the immense difficulties presented by investigation of natural phenomena." It is evident that some are more fallible than others. It is also evident that some branches of medical research offer more difficulty than others in avoiding fallibility.

Knowledge essential for effective clinical practice has not been easy to acquire. Only patients can instruct physicians; but where observations cannot be made on patients, recourse must be had to studies on other species. Such studies are based on animals living free in nature or, more usually, restricted in captivity. The overwhelming majority of the studies are artifactual, particularly when carried out on caged mammals. The studies involve inducing infections, toxic states, or nutritional disorders under conditions presumed to resemble those that occur in human disease, but they clearly never resemble them closely.

Although today we consider bedside teaching essential, there was no formal clinical teaching anywhere on the European continent, except at Leiden, until 1745. In that year (many of the Leiden faculty had moved to Vienna), ward rounds were begun in Vienna under van Swieten. Kanilfeld began this kind of teaching at Pavia in 1780, von Plenciz at Prague in 1781, Frank at Gottingen in 1784, and Hufeland at Jena in 1793. De Rechefort, who should be remembered for having introduced electroshock in the treatment of depression, is known for having originated clinical teaching in France around 1780. The rich early history of bedside teaching in Great Britain revolves mainly about the great hospital medical schools, starting with Guy's in 1723. Unlike the medicine throughout much of Europe, German medicine remained tied to dogmas until beyond the middle of the nineteenth century, except for the teaching by Frank at Gottingen and Hufeland at Jena.

Despite the growth of interest in bedside medicine in most of Europe, its teaching was inexact and ill-directed until the remarkable developments of the post-Napoleonic years at Paris and the corresponding period at Vienna. The discovery of percussion by Anenbrugger in Vienna and its promotion by Corvisart in France was followed by the discovery of auscultation by Laennec and the subsequent growth of physical diagnosis under the French physicians Louis, Bayle, and Andral, the last of whom brought the microscope and the chemistry laboratory into the service of bedside medicine. Physical diagnosis reached new heights a little later under Skoda in Vienna.

Despite these notable advances, clinical medicine could not develop assurance by bedside studies alone. It was not until Bichat and Cruvilhier in France, and later Rokitansky in Vienna, gave bedside observation the support of pathological anatomy that clinical medicine reached greatness. Bedside medicine and postmortem anatomy fed each other's growth and development, a symbiosis that unfortunately has been lost sight of in recent decades. (The close relation between pathology and medicine was recognized at Harvard as recently as 1912, when Henry Christian went from hospital pathologist to Hersey Professor of the Theory and Practice of Physic at Harvard and Physician-in-Chief of the Peter Bent Brigham Hospital.)

Gross pathology could not, however, establish etiology (except in trauma) and was also deficient in elucidating progressive states of disease. The development of pathological histology and bacteriology in the second half of the nineteenth century helped in these directions, for these disciplines remained basically patient oriented. Nevertheless many erroneous ideas resulted from the artifacts inherent in their use. The development of physiology and physiological chemistry, largely in Germany, also began slowly to enter the picture, but their influence on bedside medicine was for years small and their contributions were intermingled with some very stubbornly maintained erroneous theoretical formulations.

Among the interesting findings in chemistry was one made in 1903 by Winterstein, one of the great chemists of the time. He showed that there was no such thing as pure cholesterol more than a day or two old, when made pure it changed quickly to several dozen other compounds. This has been repeatedly verified since that time. A decade later the Russian Anitshkow stated that when he fed cholesterol to rabbits they developed atherosclerosis and that the dietary cholesterol caused the atherosclerosis; his report was received in some quarters with astonishment but for the most part only with indifference. This error was resurrected two decades later in the United States. Timothy Leary's monograph on atherosclerosis (Arch Pathol 17:434, 1934) praised the Russian theory and presented in its support a series of important-sounding irrelevancies, embellished with some gross errors. He wrote:

> Any metabolic agent capable of producing atherosclerosis must have been an article of diet from early times, since atherosclerosis has been found in mummies. The substancc is a necessary part of every animal cell, forming, from Starling's concept, the stable groundwork of the cell cytoplasm. As far as anyone knows no cholesterol is synthesized by the human body. All of the supply is ingested. The most urgent demands for it come at times of most rapid cell formation. Egg yolk is intended for the embryo. Milk is intended for the infant. It is interesting to note that Wells, in his "Outline of History," records that it was relatively late in the evolution of primitive man that he developed what Wells calls "the rather unnatural use of animal's milk as food." The high blood cholesterol found in pregnant women marks the mobilization of this substance for the needs of the fetus in utero. Man is the only animal that ingests eggs and milk* throughout its lifetime. Man is also the only animal, as far as is known, which dies in early life from coronary sclerosis, and which acquires atherosclerosis almost universally in advanced life.

This restatement of Anitshkow's theory evoked even less approval, if that is possible, than the first. Leary, like Anitshkow, ignored the fact that what he fed was a mixture of two or three dozen compounds and not cholesterol per se. The journalistic tone of his concluding statements and his grossly

*The popularity of milk is far from new. It should be remembered, for instance, that Clement of Alexandria (third century A.D.) called the Christians *galaktophogoi*. For a discussion of the symbolism of milk in Christian dogma, see Eisler, R. Orpheus the Fisher. London: Watckins, 1921, p. 62 et seq. [footnote added].

inadequate understanding of nutrition and biochemistry evoked scorn as often as indifference.

We know that much of the cholesterol in the blood and tissues is synthesized in the body, some of it in the blood vessels themselves. Today we also know that cholesterol purified every day before being administered to animals does not cause atherosclerosis and that oxides that form when cholesterol is exposed to air for a time do. The recent review by Mann (N Eng J Med 297:644-650, 1977) should dispose of the diet-cholesterol theory of atherosclerosis. It probably will not; the "mysterious viability of error" commented on by Francis Bacon in 1605 can be counted on to prevail in official dicta for years to come. The notion has become a petrifact, a word used by Spengler to describe stubbornly defended error. It may never be demolished, however strong the evidence against it. The petrifact has continually received vociferous support in irresponsible statements by journalists and spokespeople for foundations and official agencies. These statements maintain that high dietary cholesterol intakes in the industrialized nations have initiated an explosive worldwide epidemic of heart disease. Statements of this sort are reprehensible (however, unintentionally so). Although the number of cases of coronary heart disease has increased in this century, A. E. Harper (J Nutr Ed 9:154, 1977) has shown that when the statistics are corrected for the aging of the population, there has been no increase in the disease. In fact, there has been a steady decrease that started long before significant numbers of the susceptible population began to be concerned about the notion that cholesterol in the diet causes atherosclerosis.

How can errors due to indifference to artifactual factors be avoided? History provides the answer to this question. Physicians since the time of Bonet and, more strikingly, of Morgagni have used postmortem examination of their patients as a first step in clinical investigations because the examination of patients dead reveals more than the examination of patients living. Meyer Texon has used this approach and thereby provided us with a mass of unselected postmortem material on the subject. The demonstrated occurrence of the atherosclerotic lesions at bends, branchings, bifurcations, and fixed points of arteries—all areas of distorted blood flow—calls attention to the primary role of hemodynamic factors in the genesis of atherosclerosis. (An observant naturalist might have reached the same conclusion, having been struck by the fact that the only place the pike develops significant atherosclerosis is at a bend of 135° in its aorta. This experiment of nature should not have been so long ignored.) Although the ways in which hemodynamic forces stimulate the smooth muscle cells of the media to increase in number, rearrange themselves, and migrate remain incompletely defined, it must be concluded that the development of atherosclerosis is a hemodynamic phenomenon. The next step, already initiated by Texon, is the experimental production of atheroclerosis in various species according to the principles expanded in this book. After that, attempts can be made to mitigate these effects.

Meyer Texon's book, as a nonartifactual study of human atherosclerosis, stands out as a basic text of all research on the subject.

Mark D. Altschule, M.D.
Harvard Medical School

PREFACE

In 1954 I wrote a book entitled *Heart Disease and Industry* (Texon, 1954), which consisted of my clinical experience with 100 consecutive workmen's compensation cases of individuals who claimed that their heart disease was related in a causative sense to industrial conditions or incidents as described. In 78 of the 100 cases the diagnosis included arteriosclerotic heart disease due to coronary atherosclerosis (Texon, 1959). After critical analysis of the pertinent factors and findings in these cases, I concluded that coronary atherosclerosis occurs in the working population in the same manner that it occurs in the entire population.

The compelling conclusions were also drawn that the radix malorum is atherosclerosis which frequently pursues its natural course to produce myocardial infarction as a result of progressive coronary occlusive atherosclerotic disease, and that atherosclerosis is not significantly influenced by external factors such as rest, exertion, emotional stress, or nonpenetrating chest trauma. I recommended that a nonoccupational accident and sickness disability benefits insurance law be applied to heart disease so that all questions of time, place, and causal relation could be eliminated (Burchell, 1966). In 1954, after presenting a paper on heart disease and industry at the Second World Congress of Cardiology and the American Heart Association in Washington, D.C., I was invited by Dr. Paul D. White to become a member of the Committee on the Effect of Strain and Trauma on the Heart and Great Vessels of the American Heart Association, serving as a member of the subcommittee on physiology and pathology. In order to study coronary heart disease firsthand, I became a member of the Department of Forensic Medicine at the New York University Medical Center and an Assistant Medical Examiner of the City of New York, under the direction of Dr. Milton Helpern, the late Professor and Chairman of the Department of Forensic Medicine and Chief Medical Examiner of the City of New York.

My duties as a Medical Examiner included investigations at the scene of death in the many and varied circumstances that come under the jurisdiction of the Medical Examiner's office. My duties also included the pathological examination of hearts and coronary arteries of individuals of all ages who had died of heart disease as well as those who had died of other causes. I visited the laboratories of Dr. Stanley Durlacher in New Orleans and Dr. James Paterson in London, Ontario to observe their methods of tissue preparation and examination. I spent long sessions in discussions with Dr. Paul D. White, Dr. Howard Sprague, and others on the committee. My studies at the autopsy table included blood vessels in all areas of the circulation–gross observations, microscopic sections, innumerable serial sections, varied histological staining techniques, and photographs of both gross and microscopic specimens. The basic pathological findings in the atherosclerotic lesions were identified as progressing from the earliest intimal thickening to the occlusive plaque, including the variations resulting from fibroblastic proliferation, lipids, intramural hemorrhage, and thrombosis.

In pondering the bewildering mass of clinical and pathological data (Rindfleisch, 1872), I found atherosclerosis in both men and women, in relatively young as well as elderly persons, in hypertensive as well as normotensive persons (Moyer, 1971), and in lean as well as obese individuals. Notwithstanding available studies of the statistical association of atherosclerosis with lipids, diet, age, sex, hypertension (Brest and Moyer, 1974), race, occupation, smoking (Astrup and Kjeldsen, 1974), nutritional status, trace elements, enzyme systems (Zemplenyi, 1974), hormones, and emotional stress, my data indicated that the causal relation of these factors, either singly or in any combination, to atherosclerosis was not thereby proved or demonstrated. A statistical association per se does not constitute scientific proof of a causative mechanism. I became convinced that the primary causative factor or mechanism for atherosclerosis is a common denominator operating in all cases and that it determines the presence as well as the absence of atherosclerosis in all cases and in any given case.

In the fall of 1955, all the parts of the puzzle fell into place when I attempted to explain the localization of the atherosclerotic plaque. I returned to the autopsy specimens and reviewed my data from the standpoint of the laws of fluid mechanics in relation to the forces generated by flood flow, with emphasis on the biologic response of vessels with various geometric vascular configurations and different patterns of blood flow.

The puzzle was solved. I found that atherosclerosis occurs at the segmental zones of diminished lateral pressure produced by the forces generated by the flowing blood. I accumulated more specimens to demonstrate the lesions at zones of curvature, branching, bifurcation, tapering, and external attachment. In December 1955, after completing the routine autopsy work of the day, I presented my findings to Dr. Helpern and the staff at an informal conference. I emphasized and demonstrated the hydraulic conditions and the basic laws of fluid mechanics that are relevant to the development of atherosclerosis. I was encouraged to continue accumulating more specimens and anatomical proof for the hemodynamic basis of atherosclerosis. In April 1957 I presented the concept in the Ether Dome of the Massachusetts General Hospital at Medical Grand Rounds with an introduction by Dr. White. The first publication (Texon, 1957) appeared in March 1957. In 1958 the research was awarded the Hektoen Silver Medal of the American Medical Association for an exhibit at the annual meeting held in San Francisco.

The relation of the laws of fluid mechanics to human circulation and in particular to the development of atherosclerosis was becoming increasingly apparent. I consulted with Dr. Richard Skalak, James Kip Finch Professor of engineering mechanics and Chairman of the Department of Civil Engineering and Engineering Mechanics at Columbia University. Mathematical analysis of blood flow and computer studies of velocity, wall pressure, and wall shear stress were instituted for various patterns of flow. Localized areas of diminished lateral pressure in the theoretical models uniformly correlated with the localization of atherosclerotic lesions found in the human circulatory system.

It occurred to me that if a normally straight vessel were altered to become a curvature with other conditions held constant, additional support for the hemodynamic basis of atherosclerosis could be achieved. I then consulted with Dr. André Cournand and was referred to Dr. Jere R. Lord, Jr., who in turn referred me to Dr. Anthony M. Imparato. The surgical competence of Dr. Imparato led to a series of experiments in which atherosclerotic changes were produced in dogs by surgical alteration of their vascular configurations.

The hemodynamic basis of atherosclerosis has become a subject for reports, papers, chapters, meetings, and symposia both in this country and abroad. This book is the record and product of my research effort in identifying the effect of the laws of fluid mechanics as the primary causative factor in the development of atherosclerosis.

Meyer Texon

ACKNOWLEDGMENTS

In the preparation of this book, I have received help from many sources. It is a pleasure to acknowledge the initial research grant-in-aid of the National Heart Institute in 1958 (H-3590). I wish to express my sincerest thanks and gratitude to The Fan Fox and Leslie R. Samuels Foundation for the major financial support of this work by establishing The Fan Fox and Leslie R. Samuels Cardiovascular and Hemodynamics Laboratory in the Department of Forensic Medicine at the New York University Medical Center. In this laboratory additional pathological findings and correlations confirmed the original work and led ultimately to the publication of this volume. Additional financial aid in support of this research effort was provided by the Swift Newton Research Fund, the Dr. and Mrs. Henry Raphael Gold Research Fund, the Metzger-Price Research Fund, the Alan W. and Therma E. Jones Research Fund, the Emanuel Frank Foundation, the Mark Lipsky Research Fund, and the Harry A. Kurnitz Research Fund.

I am especially appreciative of the encouragement and help I received from the late Dr. Milton Helpern, Professor of Forensic Medicine at New York University Medical Center and Chief Medical Examiner of the City of New York, who witnessed the beginnings of this research effort and generously provided source material and advice. Because he was a recognized authority in pathology, his scientific endorsement and agreement with my findings were most supportive. I am deeply indebted to Anthony M. Imparato, M.D., Professor of Surgery at New York University Medical Center, for his cooperation in the experimental dog preparations. His surgical competence in altering vascular configurations provided a basic scientific support for causally relating blood flow patterns to the localization of atherosclerotic lesions.

To Richard Skalak, Chairman and James Kip Finch Professor of Civil Engineering and Engineering Mechanics at Columbia University, I express my warmest thanks for his deep interest and help by applying his expertise in fluid mechanics, computer science, and mathematical analysis to identify various patterns of flow with respect to velocity, shear stress, and wall pressure. My glass model hydraulic systems and pathological specimens provided data that uniformly correlated with his theoretical mathematical computations.

To Mark D. Altschule, M.D., Professor Emeritus of Medicine at Harvard Medical School, I owe a great deal. His rare combination of wisdom, satire, and wit pervaded many discussions we held regarding this research. From the outset we agreed that scientific truth must be stated without equivocation and without regard to its effect upon any interested parties.

To my colleagues Dr. Yong-Myun Rho, Deputy Chief Medical Examiner, Dr. Dominick J. DiMaio, Chief Medical Examiner, retired, and Dr. Elliot M. Gross, Chief Medical Examiner of the City of New York, as well as Dr. Sidney Weinberg, Chief Medical Examiner of Suffolk County, I want to express my sincere thanks for their cooperation and encouragement, especially while the data from human pathological specimens, glass hydraulic models, and experimental vascular preparations in dogs were being correlated in my hemodynamics laboratory.

For the scientific line drawings, I am indebted and deeply obligated to the late Sol Nodel who graciously applied his talent as an artist and illuminator. To my sister Frances C. Texon, who passed away while this book was in its later stages of completion, I owe thanks for her many expressions of devotion. She continued in the family tradition of solidarity and encouragement fostered by my late parents Morris David Texon and Eva Texon.

Mary Cabibbo, my secretary, deserves special thanks for her invaluable help, diligent efforts, and devotion. She not only typed the many drafts and the original manuscript of this book but also tended to the myriad of secretarial details at every stage of my research, lecturing, and publications over the many years, while at the same time helping me in my busy practice of medicine and cardiology.

To my beloved wife, Ami, who shared in all the problems that beset a practicing physician and researcher, I express thanks and deep gratitude that can hardly compensate for her love, patience, understanding, tolerance, unfailing encouragement, and sustained interest during the more than two decades of research effort that culminated in this publication.

Finally, I want to thank the publishers for their many courtesies and wholehearted cooperation.

Meyer Texon

HEMODYNAMIC BASIS OF ATHEROSCLEROSIS

1 INTRODUCTION

Modern medicine uses basic scientific facts established by many disciplines. Physicists, chemists, and engineers have frequently applied their special knowledge to medical research and have thus contributed to advances in clinical medicine. This crossing of lines that arbitrarily divide the sciences enriches both the donor and recipient disciplines. Such a cross-fertilization occurs when the laws of fluid mechanics are applied to the natural conditions in the circulatory system and to the nature and development of atherosclerosis.

Application of the laws of fluid mechanics to the natural conditions in the circulatory system reveals a rational and demonstrable basis for the localization, inception, and progressive development of atherosclerosis. Atherosclerosis does not occur at random locations. It occurs uniformly at specific sites of predilection that can be precisely defined, predicted, and produced by applying the principles of fluid mechanics. The areas of predilection for atherosclerosis are consistently found to be the segmental zones of diminished lateral pressure produced by the forces generated by the flowing blood. Such segmental zones of diminished lateral pressure are characterized by curvature, branching, bifurcation, tapering, or external attachment. Although these anatomic configurations occur in many variations of geometry, their common feature is a pattern of blood flow conducive to the production of localized areas of diminished lateral pressure. This is the initial stimulus. Atherosclerosis may therefore be considered the reactive biologic response of blood vessels to the effect of the laws of fluid mechanics, namely, the diminished lateral pressure generated by the flowing blood at sites of predilection determined by local hydraulic specifications in the circulatory system.

Research reports from this laboratory beginning in 1957 have described the prerequisite hydraulic conditions and the basic laws of fluid mechanics that are relevant to the development of atherosclerosis in the circulatory system (Texon, 1957, 1967). The hemodynamic mechanism for the localization, inception, and progressive pathological changes that characterize atherosclerotic lesions has also been described (Texon, 1963). Similarly, characteristics of blood flow in arteries (Rubinow and Keller, 1966), flow patterns, and certain theoretical calculations have been identified (Fry, 1969; Reemtsma et al., 1970; Texon, 1971). In addition, hemodynamically induced atherosclerotic lesions in dogs have been produced by the surgical alteration of vascular configurations under controlled conditions (Gyurko and Szabo, 1969; Imparato et al., 1961; Texon et al., 1962). The naturally and experimentally produced lesions in dogs and the naturally occurring lesions in humans have been illustrated and analyzed both pathologically and mathematically (Texon, 1972, 1976). The atherosclerotic changes are demonstrated consistently to result from the same specific stimulus—the diminished lateral pressure—as determined and produced by the characteristics of flowing blood and the local hydraulic specifications.

Variations as well as similarities in the severity of atheroslcerosis in different individuals and in different locations in the circulatory system of the same individual are principally caused by differences as well as similarities in local hydraulic specifications (Texon, 1974). The velocity and pattern of blood flow, the caliber of the lumen, and the anatomic configuration are of importance. A biologic factor must also be considered, namely, the local reparative reaction or pathophysiological response of the intima to the diminished lateral pressure generated by the flowing blood. It is here that the nature and degree of atherosclerotic change may be modified or influenced by differences in tissue structure and differences in cellular response arising from genetic and species characteristics (Texon, 1974).

The roles of associated or contributory factors (Werko, 1976) such as age, sex, race (Keys, 1970; Robertson et al., 1977a,b; Tillotson et al., 1973), heredity, diet (Yudkin, 1957), nutritional status, habitus, lipid metabolism (Roberts et al., 1970, 1973), cholesterol (Billings, 1962; Garrett et al., 1964; Page, 1977; Talbott, 1961), obesity, drugs, trace elements (Schroeder, 1974), associated diseases, enzyme systems (Zemplenyi et al., 1963), hormones, hypertension (Hollander, 1976; Oberman et al., 1969), occupation, and emotional stress (Friedman and Rosenman,

1974; Friedman et al., 1973) require reevaluation as secondary or modifying factors. Not one of these factors is always present (Rosenman and Friedman, 1971); nor is any particular combination present as a common denominator, *sine qua non*, or as a primary factor responsible for causing atherosclerosis. None of these factors can create or cause atherosclerosis. Atherosclerosis is found in both men and women, in the relatively young and in the elderly, in hypertensive (Kannel et al., 1976; Moser and Goldman, 1967) as well as in normotensive persons, and in learn as well as in obese individuals. Notwithstanding available studies of the statistical association of atherosclerosis with lipids (Fredrickson et al., 1967; Kannel and Gordon, 1971), diet age, sex, race, occupation (Stamler et al., 1960), hypertension (Chapman and Massey, 1964; Pickering, 1974), smoking, and emotional stress (Jenkins, 1971; Russek, 1967), proof of the causal relation of these factors (Corday and Corday, 1975; McMichael, 1976) to atherosclerosis is not thereby proved or demonstrated. A statistical association per se does not constitute scientific proof of a causative mechanism. A primary causative factor or mechanism for atherosclerosis must be a common denominator operating in all cases so that it determines the presence as well as the absence of atherosclerosis in every case.

The mechanical factors involved in atherosclerosis can be more easily defined. The localized decrease in static pressure at zones of predilection produces, in effect, a local suction action or tensile stress upon the intima at some phase of pulsatile flow in the cardiac cycle. The intima is subjected to the lifting or pulling effect of the flowing blood upon the endothelium and subjacent cells. The response is a local biologic change, a reparative or reactive thickening which results from the proliferation of endothelial cells (Altschul, 1954, Haust, 1976), fibroblasts and smooth muscle cells.

With continuing blood flow, progressive changes occur *in situ* (Duguid and Robertson, 1957). These may include elastic tissue changes, cellular infiltration, collagen deposition, lipid changes, calcification, and vascularization. The pathological processes inherent in atherosclerosis may be stationary for long periods of time or slowly progressive. Relatively quick or sudden changes (Friedman et al., 1973) may also occur. Ulceration of an atherosclerotic plaque may result from lifting off or shearing off of the superficial layers. Blood elements (Mustard and Packham, 1975) may form a thrombus at the raw or ulcerated surface. The thrombus (Spaet et al., 1974) may enlarge to a partially occlusive or totally occlusive degree by the accretion of additional blood elements. The progressive pathological process of encroachment on the lumen produces occlusive changes of all degrees. These changes are the result of the biologic or cellular response to the continuing mechanical stresses at segmental zones of the intima as determined by the flowing blood and local hydraulic specifications.

In summary, all of this laboratory's data from human specimens, model hydraulic systems, the laws of fluid mechanics, and the experimental production of hemodynamically induced arterial lesions in dogs support the hemodynamic basis of atherosclerosis and compel the conclusion that the effect of the laws of fluid mechanics—vascular dynamics—is the primary causative factor in the localization, inception, and progressive development of atherosclerosis.

2 FLUID MECHANICS— HEMODYNAMICS AND VASCULAR DYNAMICS

The flow of rivers and streams in their boundaries, the flight of airplanes, insects, and birds, the movement of ships in the water or fish in the depths, and the circulation of the blood in our arteries and veins are all varied expressions of the laws of fluid mechanics. Everywhere in this domain the laws of fluid mechanics must control.

The hemodynamic basis of atherosclerosis was first developed by correlating atherosclerotic lesions found at autopsy with their anatomical localization as determined by the laws of fluid mechanics. The forces and principles involved are directly comparable to those that prevail in all hydraulic systems with due regard to the characteristics of flowing blood and the local hydraulic specifications.

The motion of fluids may be streamline or turbulent. In a streamline or laminar flow, the fluid moves in definite layers or smooth paths. In turbulent motion the fluid moves in an eddying mass, and at a given point the velocity varies irregularly from instant to instant. At a low velocity the motion of fluid is usually laminar. As the velocity increases the laminar motion breaks down and becomes turbulent (Stehbens, 1960). Because blood flow is laminar or streamline in all the smaller blood vessels, their pressure-flow relations can be analyzed with considerable mathematical precision. In the larger arteries, some turbulence exists, and some differences from laminar flow may be expected. However, the significant features of low pressure areas occur in both laminar and turbulent flow.

When lines of flow converge there is a tendency toward stability or streamline flow. Flow in tubes with converging boundaries or narrowed lumina is characterized by an increase in velocity and a decrease in static or lateral pressure (Schultz, 1972). The decrease in lateral pressure is predictable in an inviscid fluid on the basis of Bernoulli's theorem, which states that the sum of the pressure and the square of the velocity times $\rho/2$ is constant for any two points of flow on the same streamline

$$P_1 + \tfrac{1}{2}\rho V_1^2 = P_2 + \tfrac{1}{2}\rho V_2^2 \tag{1}$$

The effect of gravity is neglected in this equation since gravity is not expected to have any significant influence on the distribution of the reduction in local pressure referred to in this presentation.

Regions of low pressure can readily be identified in a variety of local situations (Figures 1, 2, 3, 4, and 5):

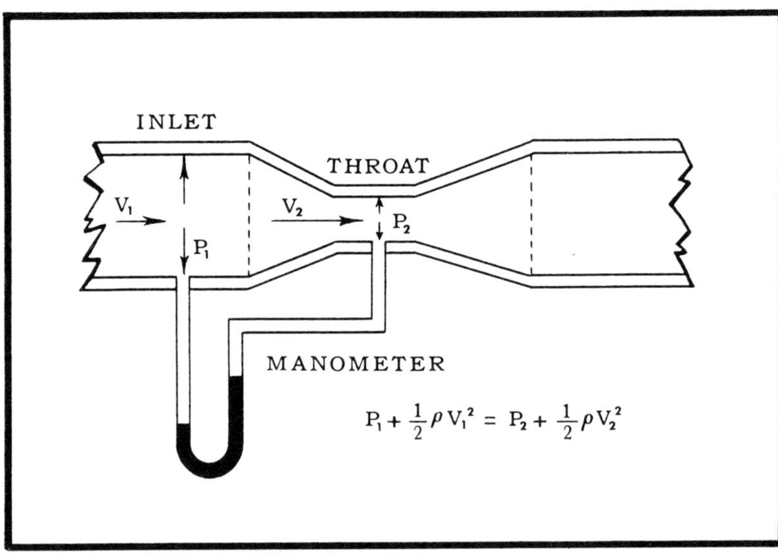

FIGURE 1. Venturi meter and Bernoulli's equation. Flow in a tube with converging boundaries causes the lateral pressure to be reduced at the narrow portion where the velocity is increased. Bernoulli's theorem states that the sum of the pressure and the square of the velocity times $\rho/2$ is constant if fluid flows from point 1 to point 2 on the same streamline. From Texon (1957). Copyright 1957, American Medical Association.

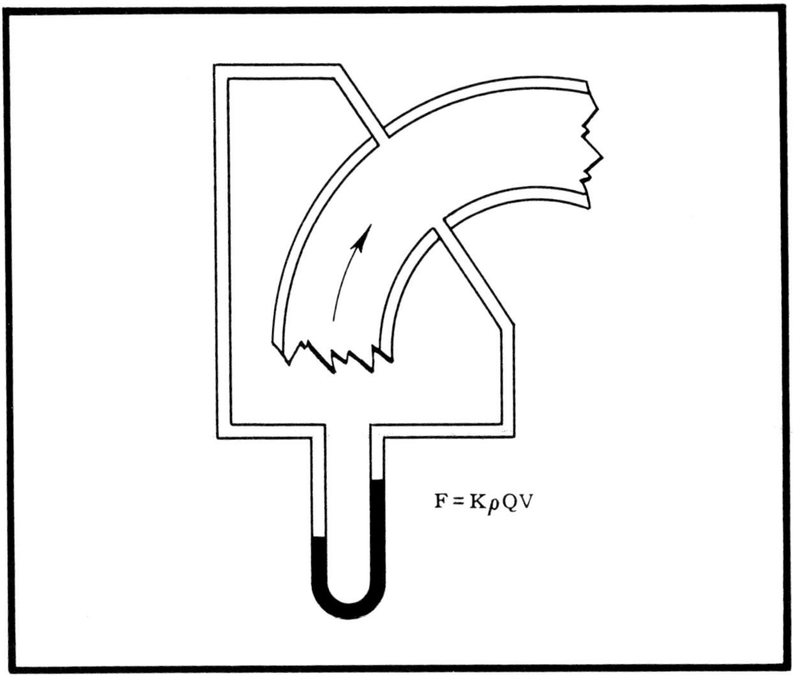

FIGURE 2. Elbow flow meter and force equation. In curvilinear motion, the lateral pressure is increased along the outer wall and decreased along the inner wall, owing to the effective centrifugal force. From Texon (1957). Copyright 1957, American Medical Association.

1. Fluid in a venturi meter, as in a tube or vessel with converging boundaries, causes the lateral pressure to be reduced at the narrow portion where the velocity is increased.
2. In curvilinear motion the lateral pressure is increased along the outer wall and decreased along the inner (convex) wall by virtue of the effective centrifugal force.
3. The velocity of flow at a cross section of tube increases from the wall toward the center. Division of the stream at a site of bifurcation results in a relative increase in velocity and a decrease in lateral pressure at the medial walls due to the local curvatures required of the streamlines.
4. At areas of external attachment, a relative diminution in lateral pressure is developed by the fixation that resists any tendency of the flowing blood to move the wall of the vessel inward toward the more central streamlines.
5. At sites of branching, the flow patterns vary but tend to develop a low pressure region on the proximal wall of the

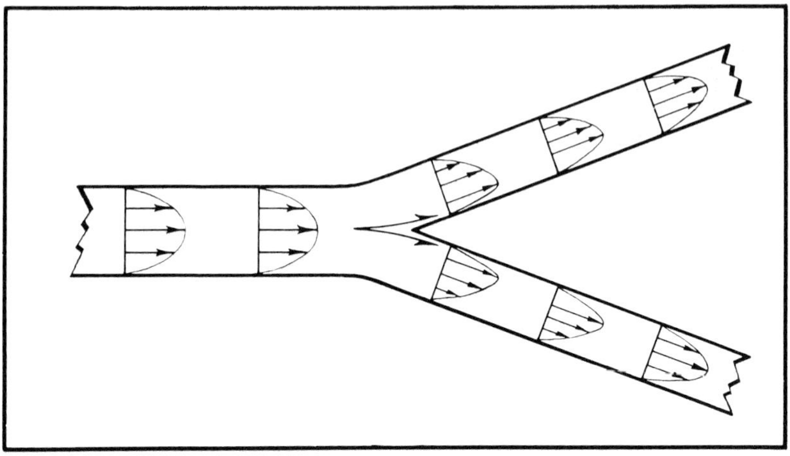

FIGURE 3. Velocity distribution for streamline flow along a tube and bifurcation. The velocity of flow at a cross section of a tube increases from the wall toward the center. Division of the axial stream results in a relative increase in velocity near the wall just downstream of the bifurcation due to the local curvatures required of the streamlines. From Texon et al. (1960). Copyright 1960, American Medical Association.

branch and distal wall of the main stem. The zones of low pressure in a branching pattern are determined by the local hydraulic specifications, which include velocity of flow, angle of branching, ratio of diameter of main stem to diameter of branch, and shape of the ostial orifice.

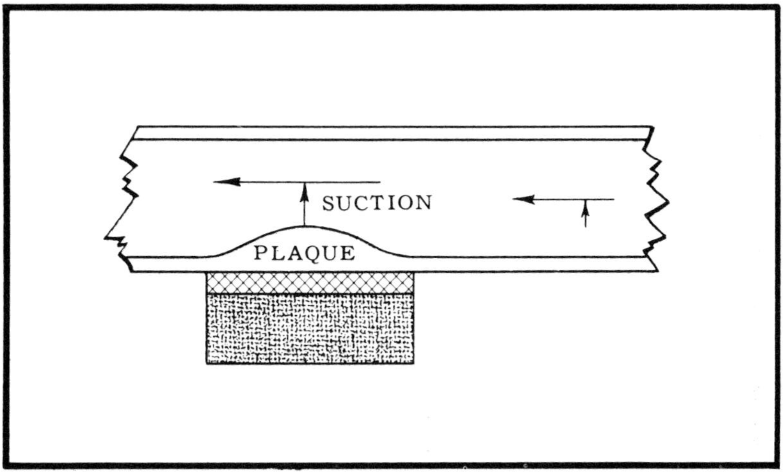

FIGURE 4. Effect of diminished lateral pressure at zone of external attachment. From Texon et al. (1963).

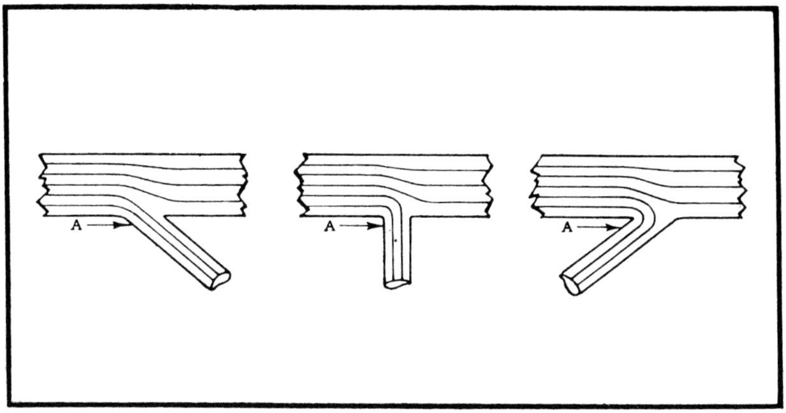

FIGURE 5. Flow patterns at sites of branching. Points "A" are low pressure areas. From Texon et al. (1963).

These anatomic patterns occur in various combinations and in many variations of geometry. In each instance low pressure zones are produced as a common feature in accordance with the laws of fluid mechanics. The sites of predilection for atherosclerosis are uniformly found to be precisely those locations characterized by a relative reduction in lateral pressure.

3 RELEVANT HYDRAULIC PARAMETERS

The distribution of pressure in any hydraulic system is determined by the composite effect of many factors. In the circulatory system the relevant parameters include the following:

I. Physical characteristics of the blood
   A. Viscosity, μ (centipoise, cp)
   B. Specific gravity, S, or density, ρ (g/cm^3)
   C. Homogeneity
   D. Particulate content and hematocrit
   E. Temperature

II. Flow characteristics
   A. Velocity of flow, V (cm/s)
   B. Pressure, P (dyn/cm^2)
   C. Volumetric rate of flow, Q (cm^3/s)
   D. Pulsation of flow
   E. Pulse rate, rhythm, and amplitude
   F. Reynolds number, $\mathrm{Re} = VD\rho/\mu$
   G. Shear stress

III. Anatomic pattern (Geometry)
   A. Caliber of lumen, D (cm)
   B. Bifurcation
   C. Tapering
   D. Branching characteristics
   E. Curvature
   F. Total area of flow

IV. Fabric or local mural factors
   A. External attachment
   B. External pressure
   C. Thickness
   D. Elasticity
   E. Porosity
   F. Strength of bond between layers

4 SITES OF PREDILECTION OR LOCALIZATION AND THE MECHANISM FOR INCEPTION AND PROGRESSIVE CHANGES

The pressure difference between the outside and the inside of the wall of a blood vessel is the net force per unit area exerted on the wall that tends to move the wall of the blood vessel. For a given geometry of curve, taper, bifurcation, branch, or attachment, the maximum pressure difference is a function of the Reynolds number of the flow and is proportional to ρV^2 where ρ is the density and V is the velocity. A localized decrease in static pressure at points of predilection produces, in effect, a local suction action upon the wall. The intima is here subjected to the lifting or pulling effect of the flowing blood upon the endothelial layer and subjacent cells. This force is the initial stimulus. The initial response is a local biologic change, a reparative process or reactive thickening due to the proliferation of endothelial cells and fibroblasts from subjacent layers. There is no evidence of cellular (blood) reaction, vascularization, or lipid change in the earliest stage of intimal thickening. The endothelial and internal elastic layers appear to remain intact and unchanged in the early lesion. With continuing blood flow, the thickening intima encroaches upon the lumen (Plate 1).* The

*Color plates may be found between pages 36 and 37.

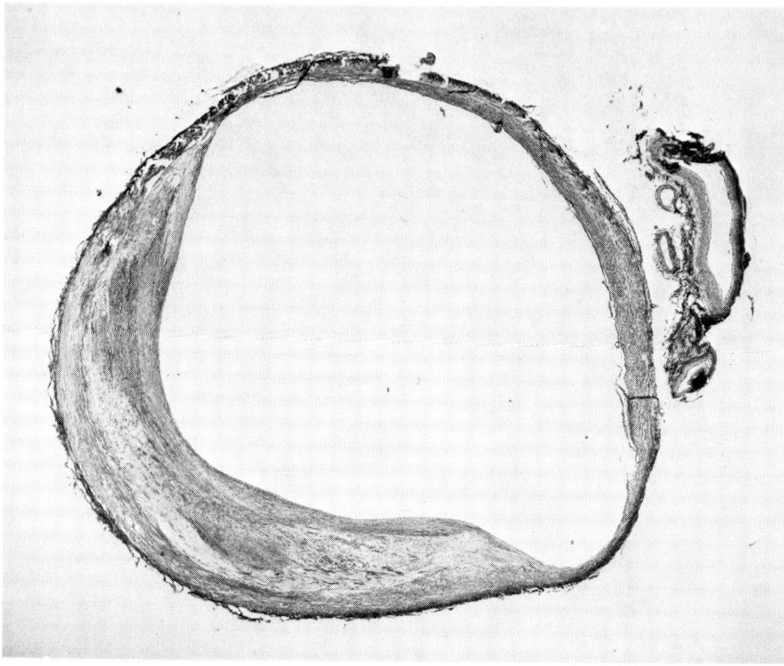

FIGURE 6. White woman, age 65, internal carotid artery–showing eccentric atherosclerotic plaque in a "curvature" lesion. Layers of intimal fibroblastic proliferation reflect the orientation of cells to successive hydraulic forces. From Texon (1967).

lateral pressure becomes further reduced as the caliber of the lumen diminishes. The plaque assumes characteristics of shape and degrees of further pathological change that correspond to zones of varying diminution in lateral pressure. The orientation of cells to successive hydraulic forces is manifested by the successive layers of fibroblastic proliferation (Figure 6) that appear as the dominant pathological change at all stages. Cellular (blood) elements and lipids may be added to the intimal fibroblastic proliferation as part of the pathological change *in situ*. The earliest lipid change is noted as droplets within smooth muscle cells or fibroblasts in the basement zone of the intimal plaque (Plate 2). More advanced lesions (Stehbens, 1974) reveal free lipid droplets that coalesce and extend toward the luminal surface subjacent to the plaque's fibrous cap. In some lesions the intimal proliferation extends across the lumen as tongue-like projections producing a multi-luminal channel (Figures 7 and 8). The growth and direction of such tongue-like lesions are influenced by the hydraulic forces present, especially velocity of flow. Vascularization and hemorrhage within an intimal plaque have been observed (Plate 3). Advanced lesions may be partially or completely occlusive (Plate 4) and consist of layered fibroblastic proliferation with combined evidences of old hemorrhage, fatty change, and cellular proliferation.

The atherosclerotic plaque, which begins as a minute reactive thickening due to proliferation of endothelial cells and fibroblasts at sites of diminished lateral pressure in the circulatory system, evolves through progressive stages (Wissler and Geer, 1972) that vary in their rate of development as well as in the nature, extent, and complexity of pathological change. These are *in situ* pathological processes that may include elastic tissue changes, collagen deposition, fibrosis, cellular infiltration, lipid

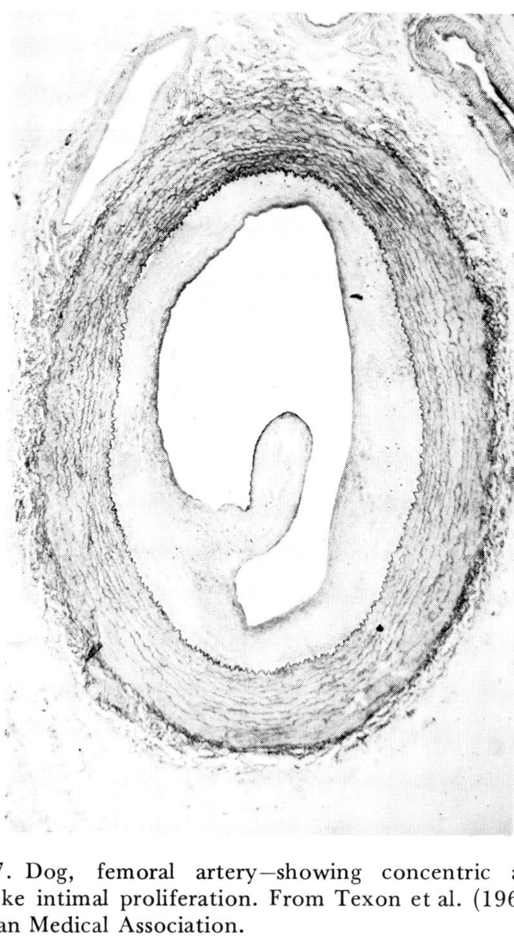

FIGURE 7. Dog, femoral artery—showing concentric atherosclerosis with tongue-like intimal proliferation. From Texon et al. (1965). Copyright 1965, American Medical Association.

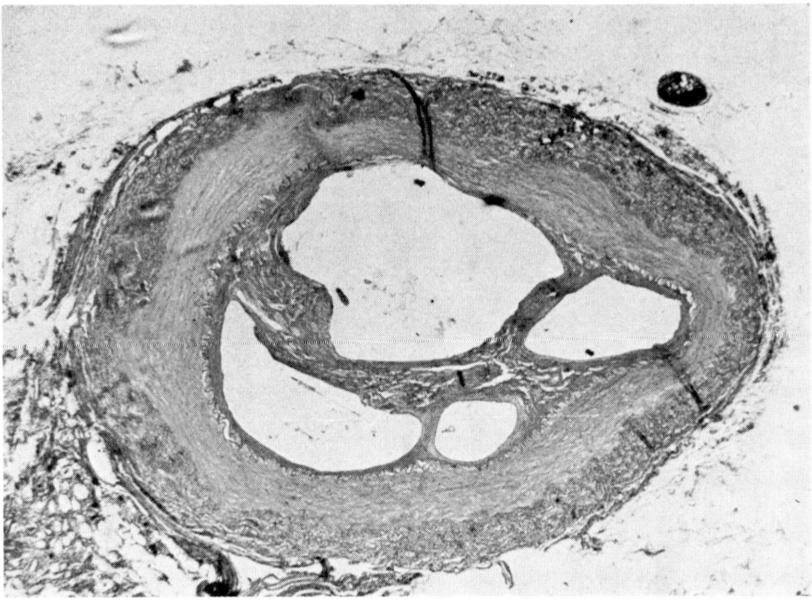

FIGURE 8. Dog No. 2134, femoral artery—intimal proliferation subdivides the lumen at site of suture attachment. From Texon et al. (1965). Copyright 1965, American Medical Association.

changes, and occasional calcification. Vascularization of the plaque may also occur by growth of capillaries from the adventitia or, more rarely, from the lumen.

The continuous operation of local hydraulic factors makes progressive pathological changes inherently possible. The pathological process may be relatively stationary for long periods, slowly progressive, or episodic. A critical stage in the pathogenesis may arrive when a quick or dramatic change occurs. The superficial layers of an atherosclerotic plaque may become ruptured, lifted, or sheared off (Figure 9). The atheromatous content of the plaque is drawn into the blood stream and embolized distally. A raw or ulcerated surface is exposed to the flowing blood elements (Mustard and Packham, 1970, 1975) These may become deposited or adherent to the plaque to form a thrombus. The thrombus may enlarge to a partially or totally occlusive degree by the accretion of additional blood elements. An intramural or intimal hemorrhage may result from the same hydraulic forces that tend to draw the plaque toward the lumen. The intima is split or torn locally to produce a microscopic hemorrhage in a manner comparable to a gross medial dissecting hematoma of the aorta. Intimal hemorrhages in association with or as part of the atherosclerotic plaque are frequent. They vary in size; although a small hemorrhage may not be sufficient to affect significantly the caliber of the lumen, a large hemorrhage may reduce an already narrowed lumen to the stage of total occlusion.

The pathological process inherent in atherosclerosis produces occlusive changes of all degrees as the net result of the vascular response to local hemodynamic factors. Partial to complete occlusion may result locally from: (1) progressive intimal thickening, (2) thrombosis (Roberts and Bujor, 1972) superimposed upon the ulcerated luminal surface of an atherosclerotic plaque,

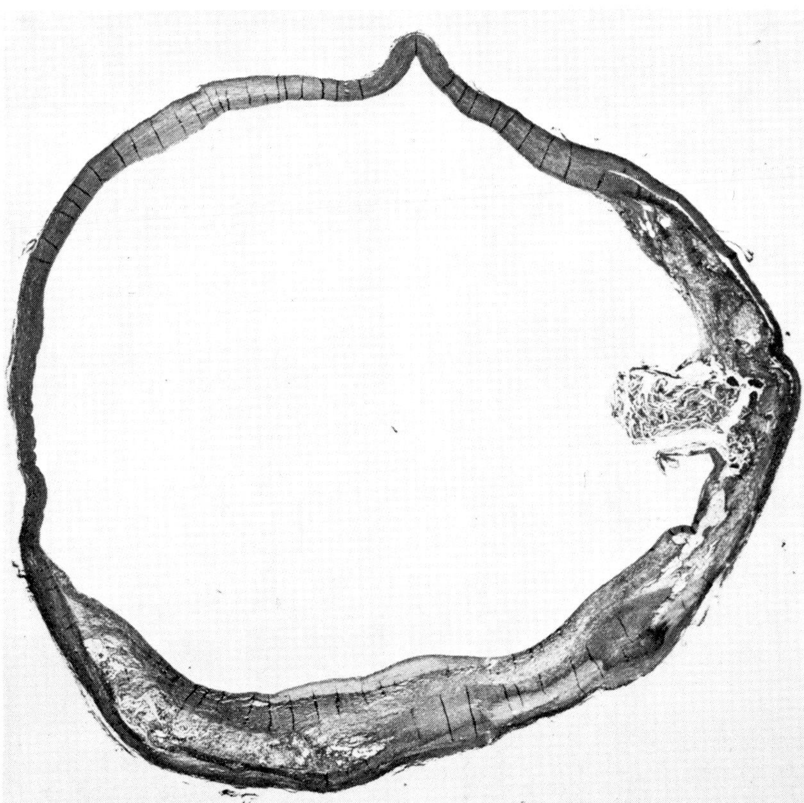

FIGURE 9. Human thoracic aorta—showing atherosclerotic plaque on dorsal wall (attachment lesion). Note rupture of superficial layers of plaque and embolization of atheromatous contents. From Texon (1957). Copyright 1957, American Medical Association.

and (3) intimal hemorrhage within or in association with an atherosclerotic plaque. While encroachment upon the lumen of a blood vessel may be due to any one or any combination of these pathological changes, the commonly encountered completely occlusive lesion is that in which the lumen is obliterated by progressive thickening of the intima with incorporated old hemorrhage in various stages of transformation.

Partial to complete distal occlusion may result from embolization of the atherosclerotic contents of a plaque by rupture of the overlying fibrous cap as it is drawn toward the axial stream.

The localization and progressive changes in naturally occurring lesions in humans are comparable to the lesions experimentally produced in dogs by the surgical alteration of vascular configurations under controlled conditions. In brief, atherosclerotic lesions, whether occurring naturally or induced by altering the hemodynamics, are consistently found at sites of diminished lateral pressure. These segmental low pressure zones are sites of predilection for atherosclerosis that derive from local hydraulic specifications.

5 BLOOD FLOW CHARACTERISTICS IN ARTERIES

Solutions of the equations of fluid mechanics have been given for steady and oscillatory flow in straight rigid tubes (Rudinger, 1966). Additional modifications of flow in the animal or human circulatory system are due to (1) the elasticity of the blood vessels (Bergel, 1961; Wormersley, 1957), (2) the pulsatile character of the flow (Davids et al., 1971), (3) the viscous properties of the blood as a suspension of particles in a colloid solution, (4) the complex ejection pattern of blood flow in the aorta, and (5) the flow pattern determined by the intricate combinations of structure or anatomic design that characterizes the arterial and venous circulation. Some simplification of the analysis of blood flow in arteries is justified here because the major hydraulic conditions that pertain to the development of atherosclerosis occur in both steady and pulsatile flow.

LAMINAR FLOW

Laminar or streamline flow in a circular tube is also called "Poiseuille flow." Poiseuille, a physician, first studied the steady flow of liquids in cylindrical tubes. Poiseuille's law states that the pressure drop is directly proportional to the length of the tube, to the rate of flow, and to the viscosity; and inversely proportional to the fourth power of the radius. If the velocity of flow is increased to a critical point the laminar motion breaks down and becomes turbulent; Poiseuille's law no longer applies. The laws governing pressure-flow relations in turbulent flow are less easily subjected to precise analysis. The transition from laminar to turbulent flow occurs at critical conditions that depend on the velocity of flow, the density and viscosity of the liquid, and the diameter of the tube. These factors are combined in the Reynolds number defined by

$$\mathrm{Re} = \frac{VD\rho}{\mu} \tag{2}$$

A Reynolds number of 2000 is usually given as the critical value for transition from laminar to turbulent flow. However, this number may vary with other conditions of flow such as varying rates of flow and disturbances in the flow. The Reynolds number for blood flow in the circulatory system, except in the larger arteries, is generally found to be well below the critical level for turbulence. In the larger arteries, despite the existence of local areas of turbulence during some part of the cardiac cycle, essentially laminar flow may be assumed for calculation of average pressure-flow relations without the introduction of any significant error.

PULSATILE FLOW

Arterial blood flow is characterized by the recurring pulsation imparted by systolic contraction of the heart (Rushmer, 1970). Pulsations modify the instantaneous pressure-flow relations found in a steady flow (Attinger, 1964; McDonald, 1974). At all frequencies of oscillatory or pulsatile flow a variable lag is produced between the applied pressure and the ensuing movement of the fluid. The laminae nearest the wall have the lowest velocity due to the effect of viscosity. The flow near the wall has relatively less kinetic energy and reverses easily with each half-cycle. In the more central streamlines the velocity and kinetic energy are greatest. With reduction in pressure gradient and reversal of flow at the half-cycle, the axial streamline may be still flowing forward when reversal of the direction of flow may be occurring in the peripheral laminae. In such conditions the average velocity may approach zero. As the frequency of pulsation increases, the axial stream's velocity is reduced and the parabolic distribution of velocity across the tube flattens.

BLOOD VISCOSITY

A precise theoretical analysis of the flow of liquids generally assumes the fluid to be homogeneous, of uniform viscosity, and a "Newtonian" fluid. Blood is not a simple fluid; it has anomalous viscous properties. In the flowing blood the relatively cell-free zone of plasma that appears close to the wall of the blood vessel causes a local decrease in viscosity. This effect becomes important in the relatively slow rate of capillary blood flow and in vessels of less than 0.5 mm in diameter (Bugliarello, 1966; Wiener et al., 1966). Under conditions of relatively high velocity, as in the arteries that develop atherosclerosis, the variable viscosity of the blood does not alter appreciably the pressure-flow calculations. In such instances, blood may be considered to behave as a Newtonian fluid. Variation in viscosity, as a physical characteristic of blood, does not appear to influence significantly the role of hemodynamics in the development of atherosclerosis.

MOVEMENT OF THE ARTERIAL WALL (ELASTICITY)

Arteries vary in diameter and length during the cardiac cycle (McDonald, 1960; Patel et al., 1964). The transient dilatation following systole is relatively small, and its effect on the stability of flow is negligible when compared with the effects of the average or peak velocity of flow. Likewise, the longitudinal movement of the arteries is usually slight because of the anatomic attachments. The behavior of the arterial wall as an elastic tube (Evans, 1962; Skalak and Stathis, 1966) affects the propagation and damping of the pulse wave (Anliker and Maxwell, 1966; Ogden, 1966; Streeter et al., 1963; Wylie, 1966) but has no appreciable effect on the average pressure-flow relationships that pertain to the development of atherosclerosis. In a larger artery, notably the arch of the aorta (Fry et al., 1957), vascular elasticity helps to produce streamline flow by reducing the pressure and velocity fluctuations throughout the cardiac cycle by its action as a surge chamber.

PRESSURE-FLOW RELATIONS

In a steady flow the rate of discharge through a tube is directly proportional to the pressure gradient in accordance with Poiseuille's law. The pressure gradient is the difference in pressure between two points in a continuous hydraulic system divided by the distance between the two points. This difference in pressure rather than the absolute values of pressure determines the velocity of flow (Gabe, 1965). Thus, if there is no difference in pressure between two points, there is no flow, regardless of the absolute pressure present. Accordingly, a reduction in the difference in pressure (gradient) will decrease the velocity of flow between two points under observation in a continuous hydraulic system (Krovetz, 1965). The chief determinants of the pressure gradient are the flow rate, the vessel diameter, and the viscosity of the fluid. A rise or fall in absolute pressure in a tube will not influence volumetric flow significantly. Similarly, the cyclic changes in absolute pressure levels of the arterial tree do not affect appreciably the flow volume. The variable pressure gradient inherent in pulsatile flow produces a variable velocity of flow (Noordergraaf et al., 1964). The peak velocity may be significantly greater than the average velocity with consequently greater effect on the development of atherosclerosis.

An equation relating volumetric flow to a varying pressure gradient may be derived by methods similar to the derivation of Poiseuille's equation (Cohen, 1964). Although steady flow rate is dependent chiefly on the magnitude of the average pressure gradient, pulsatile flow rate is dependent on the frequency of oscillation of the pulse pressure as well as its amplitude.

The arterial tree branches progressively (Pedley et al., 1971) so that the cross-sectional area of the branches generally increases peripherally. However, the total wall area of the branches, hence the friction or resistance, also increases with the number of branches and causes an increased pressure gradient. The velocity of flow is related to the total cross-sectional area of the vascular bed rather than the caliber of a single vessel. The velocity of flow in the arterial system thus generally decreases with increasing distance from the heart.

The velocity of flow may also be influenced by external pressure or arteriolar constriction. Blood flow may then cease or be directed to alternate channels.

CAVITATION

There is no evidence that the phenomenon of cavitation occurs in the circulatory system (McDonald, 1960). In fluid mechanics, cavitation occurs as a liquid flows, usually at high velocity, past a surface or through a passage when the pressure falls below vapor pressure at a particular temperature. The liquid vaporizes and a cavity or void forms. The alternate formation and collapse of the vapor bubbles is responsible for noise, reduced efficiency, and the pitting of metal parts by the intermittent pressure of high intensity on small areas. These intermittent pressures can exceed the tensile strength of many metals. Particles of metal broken out by cavitation can progressively erode and weaken even metals of high strength.

BOUNDARY LAYER

The boundary layer theory is based on the assumption that (1) close to the wall of a blood vessel (for high enough Reynolds numbers) there exists a thin layer of fluid in which the velocity gradient is large enough to produce viscous stresses of a significant magnitude and (2) in the remaining portion of the fluid outside the boundary layer, viscous forces may be neglected.

The boundary layer remains in contact with the entire surface of a body, such as an airfoil or wall of a blood vessel, provided the inclination of the surface to the direction of motion is not too great. When the angle of divergence is excessive, the boundary layer may detach itself (Gutstein et al., 1968; Schneck and Gutstein, 1966) and a surface of discontinuity forms (Figure 10). This surface of discontinuity usually rolls up into vortices and forms a wake.

Downstream of a point of separation of the boundary layer in a tube there is usually a region of increasing pressure. The pressure distribution on the surface of the body or on the wall of the channel is determined by the shape of the body or channel.

Separation of the flow from a boundary surface produces a change in velocity distribution within the boundary layer. The point of separation is a point of stagnation on that streamline that divides the oncoming flow from the reverse flow of a region of discontinuity. The change in curvature of the velocity profile is due to the adverse pressure gradient, namely, the positive gradient. The point of separation is also determined by the stage of development already attained by the boundary layer in the upstream region. A laminar boundary layer will lead to separation at an earlier point than a turbulent layer; in both cases a region of appreciable deceleration will cause separation.

In a converging channel the flow is accelerated in the converging section and some pressure head is converted to velocity head. This is a stable and efficient process with only small losses of energy and no eddy formation.

In a diverging channel the flow may be unstable if the angle

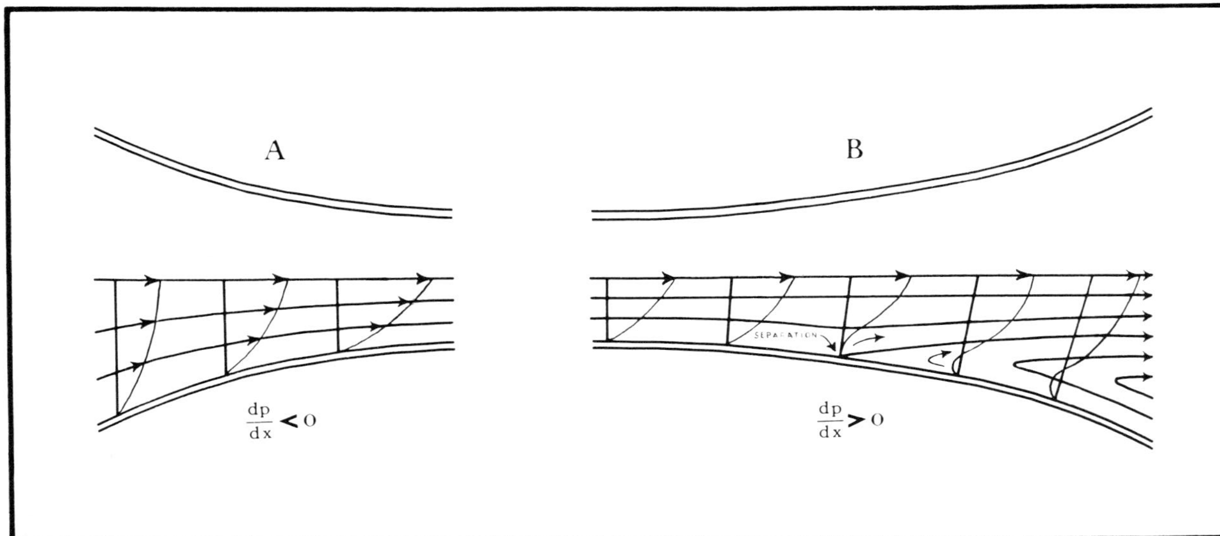

FIGURE 10. Separation of flow from a boundary surface: Effect of acceleration (A) and deceleration (B) upon velocity distribution (see text). From Texon (1971).

of divergence is considerable. Some velocity head is converted to pressure head. Some of the kinetic energy is converted to thermal energy because of the viscosity of the fluid. The fluid may not fill the channel and separation may take place, just as the stall of a lifting vane. Flow in a diverging channel is unstable and less efficient and may produce large energy losses and eddy formation.

If p is the static pressure and x is the distance along the channel, the derivative dp/dx is the pressure gradient. In a straight channel dp/dx would be zero if no friction were present. If friction were present dp/dx would be negative; there would be a pressure drop. In a converging channel dp/dx would be negative. In a diverging channel dp/dx is positive; the pressure rises along the channel. This rise in pressure may account in part for the poststenotic dilatation frequently seen in atherosclerotic vessels.

In summary, when lateral pressure decreases with acceleration, the velocity distribution becomes more uniform and stable. On the other hand, when the pressure increases with deceleration, the velocities become unequal until one eventually reaches zero velocity. At this point, separation may occur and the mainstream of the flow may leave the surface of the body or vessel wall. This results in a discontinuity of flow—but not in fluid, as in the case of cavitation—for the region of discontinuity is generally filled with fluid moving in the upstream direction along the wall.

STRESSES GENERATED BY FLOWING BLOOD

Flowing blood generates varying physical stresses (Caro et al., 1971) upon the walls of blood vessels serving as conduits for the blood (Gessner, 1973). Physical or mechanical stress is defined as a force acting per unit area of surface. The stress at any point of a surface may be resolved into a normal component acting perpendicularly to the surface and a shear component acting parallel to the surface. Normal stresses (σ) may be either tensile or compressional depending on the direction of the force with respect to the reference surface. Similarly, the effect of shear stress (τ) may produce either a tensile or compressional force with respect to the reference surface. A specific stress component is characterized by its magnitude and direction with respect to a given surface. In contrast to steady flow, which characteristically produces a relatively constant compressional or tensile stress at a given site, pulsatile flow may be characterized by alternating compressional and tensile stresses at the same site. Turbulent flow may also be characterized by stresses occurring irregularly at a given site.

The hydraulic factors that are chiefly responsible for normal stresses and shear stresses are the anatomical pattern (geometry of design) and the velocity distribution in the blood vessel. The shear stress at the wall depends on the velocity gradient (Fry, 1968) at the interface. The velocity distribution or profile, which determines the velocity gradient at the interface in various vascular configurations, can be analyzed more precisely in steady flow than in pulsatile or turbulent flow. In all patterns of flow, however, a relative decrease in lateral pressure tends to develop at certain zones of predilection, namely, curvature, branching, bifurcation, tapering, and external attachment. The decrease in lateral pressure may be related to a local increase in blood velocity. Also, an increased velocity usually leads to an increase in shear stress at the interface. In fact, shear stress, diminished lateral pressure, and tensile stress may be different expressions denoting coincidental forces at a given site.

Shear stress at the wall of a blood vessel (Figure 11) is proportional to the rate of change in velocity of the blood flow in a direction normal (perpendicular) to the wall. The slope of

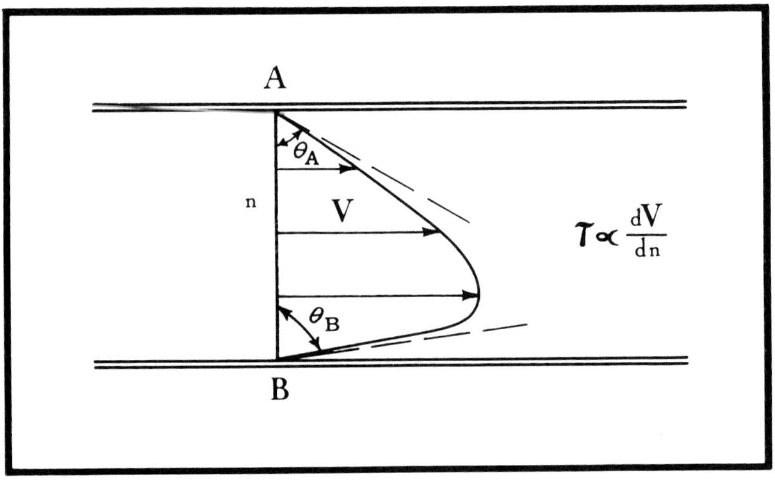

FIGURE 11. In an unsymmetric velocity profile, the shear stress at the wall in a two-dimensional flow is greater at B than at A since the shear stress is proportional to the velocity gradient, which is in turn proportional to the slope of the tangents to the velocity profile. As shown, $\theta B > \theta A$ and hence $\tau B > \tau A$. From Texon (1972).

the velocity profile away from the n axis is the value dV/dn, which is related to the shear stress (τ) on the interface. The order of magnitude of the shear stress at the wall in small blood vessels may be estimated from Poiseuille's law. For a vessel with a diameter D of 2 mm, with a mean flow velocity V of 3 cm/s and a viscosity μ of 4 cp, the shear stress at the wall is

$$\tau = \frac{8V\mu}{d} = \frac{4.8 \text{ dyn}}{\text{cm}^2} \tag{3}$$

However, because of asymmetry and bends, it is possible for local shear stress to be several times the mean value.

TURBULENCE

As shown in Figure 10, separation from a bounding surface may occur in many places where there are departures of the walls from a perfectly straight configuration. Where separated zones occur at a high Reynolds number, they contain a relatively stagnant fluid that has a general vortical motion and is also usually quite turbulent. The point of separation may also change its location rapidly and frequently. The fluctuations due to the turbulence of a moving point of separation may subject the endothelial layer of the artery to many rapid changes of shear stress and pressure. The rapid fluctuations of these stresses may possibly be the initiating agency of atherosclerotic effects. The regions of separation generally correspond to regions of low mean pressure so that the correspondence previously mentioned of regions of low pressure areas with atherogenesis may in fact be indicative of other flow characteristics that happen to be present in approximately these same areas.

DIVIDER FLOW

When a flow is divided by the ridge between two daughter vessels, the high velocity near the center of the artery does impinge on the point of bifurcation. The velocity near the wall just downstream of the bifurcation may be greater than normal near the wall (Figure 3). The pressure in the fluid is not decreased by Bernoulli's equation when this kind of division takes place, but there may be a region of decreased lateral pressure at the medial walls due to the local curvatures required of the streamlines downstream of the bifurcation. This may also lead to separated zones.

SUCTION EFFECT

In an area of diminished lateral pressure, the pressure distribution may be regarded as the full arterial pressure plus an area of negative pressure superimposed on the normal positive pressure. The absolute pressure at any point is still positive (compression). However, the change or decrement in the pressure may be regarded as a local suction pressure relative to the arterial pressure. If the wall were highly porous so that a tissue pressure in the wall might be more or less equal to mean arterial pressure, then this wall pressure might be greater in the interior of the wall than the pressure exerted by the blood in the region of the diminished lateral pressure. This difference of pressure, tissue pressure in the wall being greater than the blood pressure at the point, will have the effect of tending to push the interior layers toward the center of the lumen. Note that such effects do not involve any tensile forces but the displacement produced by the pressures would be in the direction of a displacement produced by the tensile force on the wall.

6 THEORETICAL CALCULATIONS FOR DIFFERENT FLOW PATTERNS

The forces generated by the flowing blood can be computed in certain idealized situations. The values calculated will be increasingly reliable as technologic instrumentation improves and as hydraulic specifications are more accurately defined.

TAPER

Bernoulli's equation

$$P_1 + \tfrac{1}{2}\rho V_1^2 = P_2 + \tfrac{1}{2}\rho V_2^2$$

provides a basis for computing the velocity and pressure relations in a tapering vessel. The computations must consider the effect of branch runoffs if present between the points under study. In some instances the effect of gravity may be important.

CURVATURE, BENDS, AND THE FORCE EQUATION

The total force required to deflect a steady stream of fluid through a given angle (Figure 12) is given by

$$F = K\rho QV \qquad (4)$$

where F = total force in dyn, K = coefficient (see Table 1), ρ = density in g/cm^3, Q = flow rate in cm^3, and V = velocity in

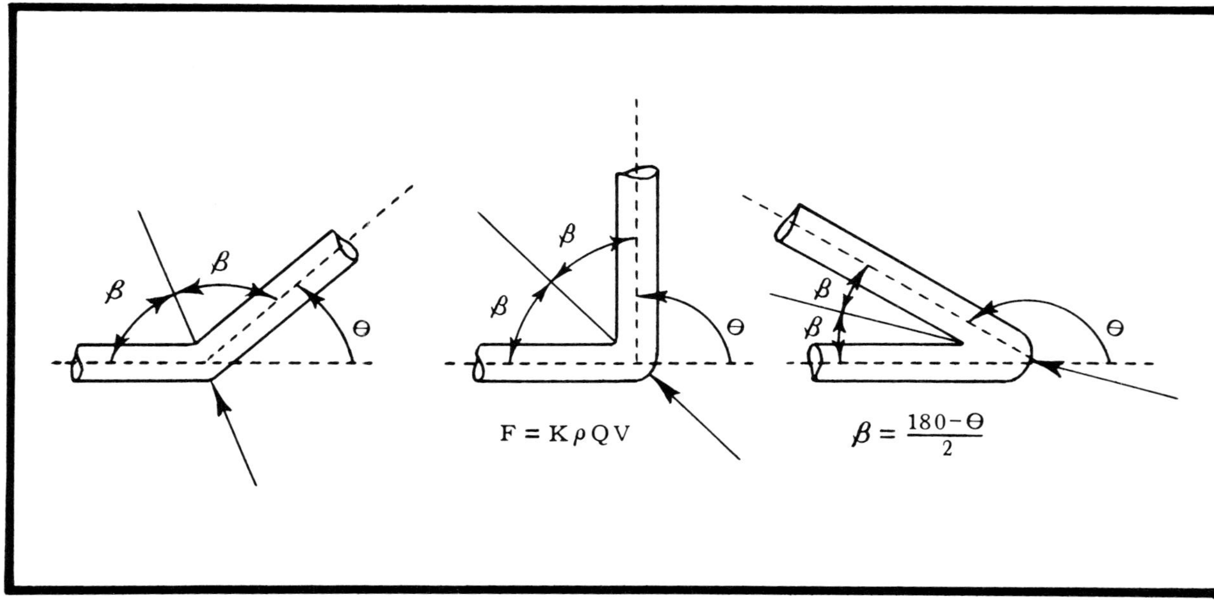

FIGURE 12. Diagrams and force equation at bends. From Texon (1963).

TABLE 1. Value of Coefficient K with Angle θ*

θ Degrees	K	θ Degrees	K
0	0	105	1.58
15	0.26	120	1.73
30	0.52	135	1.85
45	0.76	150	1.93
60	1.00	165	1.97
75	1.22	180	2.00
90	1.41	$\beta = (180 - \theta)/2$	

*See Figure 12.
Note: From Texon (1963).

cm/s. The value of the coefficient K depends on the angle θ (Table 1). If $\rho = 1$ g/cm^3, $A = 0.20$ cm^2, $V = 20$ cm/s, then $Q = AV = 4$ cm^3/s, and from the formula $F = K\rho QV$, at 45°, $F = 61$ dyn; at 90°, $F = 113$ dyn; at 135°, $F = 148$ dyn; and at 180° $F = 160$ dyn.

At a constant velocity and volumetric flow any increase in the angle θ increases the force required to divert the stream. By halving the diameter and maintaining the volumetric flow, the velocity must increase fourfold; thus, the force is increased by increasing the velocity (see Table 1).

The computation of the forces described here, it should be noted, does not describe their distribution. However, it is reasonable to assume that the net effect must be an increased pressure on the outer curvature and a decreased pressure (net suction action) on the inner curvature. It is this suction effect that evokes the atherosclerotic response.

Relation between Pressure and Radius of Curvature

Flow in a curved path (McConalogue and Spivastava, 1968) is so common in the circulatory system that special emphasis on this type of flow is appropriate (Binder, 1955).

Consider the flow of an infinitesimal element between two concentric streamlines an infinitesimal distance apart (Figure 13). The radius of curvature of this path is r, and the tangential linear velocity is V. If the height of the element is dr and the area is dA then the mass of the element is $\rho\, dr\, dA$ (mass = density × volume). The normal or radial acceleration is V^2/r. The effective centrifugal force acting on the element is the product

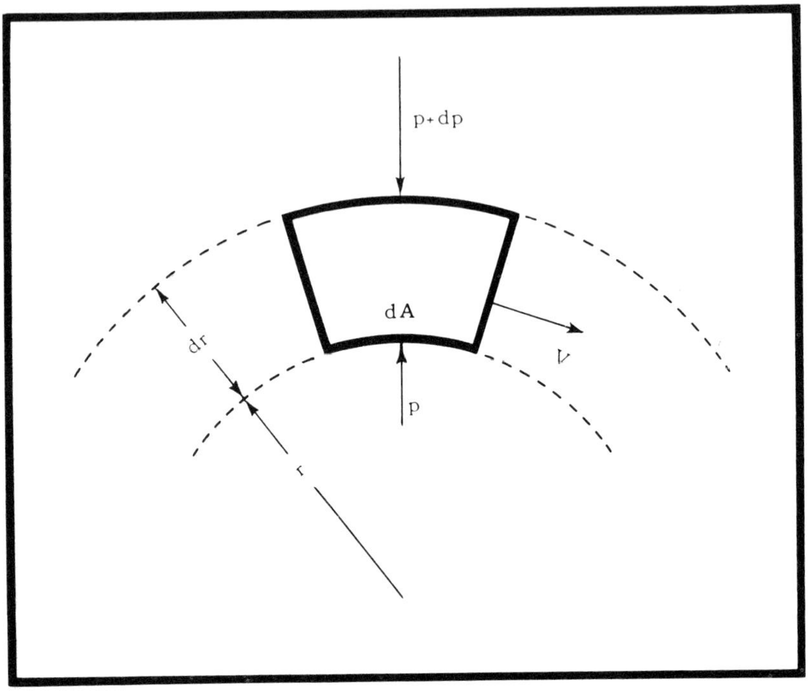

FIGURE 13. Flow in a curved path. From Texon (1967).

of mass and acceleration or $\rho\, dr\, dA\ (V^2/r)$. The pressure varies from p to $p + dp$ as the radius varies from r to $r + dr$. The effective centrifugal force on the element is balanced by the resultant forces over the surfaces. A force balance in the radial direction gives

$$dp\ dA = \rho \left(\frac{V^2}{r}\right) dr\ dA \tag{5}$$

and

$$dp = \rho \left(\frac{V^2}{r}\right) dr \tag{6}$$

The pressure increases with radius in a curved flow. There is a fall in pressure per unit radial distance toward the center of curvature by the amount $\rho V^2/r$; i.e., the pressure gradient $dp/dr = \rho V^2/r$.

While Bernoulli's equation usually applies to flow along a streamline, Eq. (6) defines the fundamental relation $dp = \rho V^2/r\ dr$, which provides a method for studying conditions in a direction normal to the streamlines. If the streamline is straight, the pressure change normal to the streamline is zero because r is infinitely large. For streamlines of finite curvature, the pressure varies from p to $\rho + dp$ in the distance dr. Since dp is positive if dr is positive, Eq. (6) shows that the pressure decreases for successive points from the concave to the convex side of the stream. The exact variation in pressure depends upon the variation in velocity with radius and the local radius of curvature of the streamlines.

The velocity distribution for certain ideal curvilinear flows is known; the case of a free vortex is illustrated (Figure 14). In this case the velocity increases as the radius decreases. In an actual flow around a bend, viscous effects, the pulsatility of the flow, and the elasticity of the wall will produce modifications of this idealized pattern. However, for any case of curved flow, the pressure will increase with the radius, and the order of magnitude can be approximated by assuming a free vortex velocity distribution. On a meteorologic scale, the low pressure found in the eye of tornadoes and hurricanes is explained on the same basis.

The pressure distribution in a free vortex can be determined by substituting the relation $V = K/r$ in the equation $dp = \rho V^2/r\,dr$ and integrating between limits. K is determined by the known velocity and radius at a particular point.

$$\int_1^2 dp = \rho \int_1^2 \frac{V^2}{r}\, dr$$

$$P_2 - P_1 = \rho K^2 \int_1^2 \frac{dr}{r^3} = \left(\frac{1}{r_1^2} - \frac{1}{r_2^2}\right) \rho \frac{K^2}{2} \tag{7}$$

Since $V_1 r_1 = V_2 r_2 = K$, the equation may be written

$$P_1 + \tfrac{1}{2}\rho V_1^2 = P_2 + \tfrac{1}{2}\rho V_2^2$$

$$\frac{P_1}{w} + \frac{V_1^2}{2g} = \frac{P_2}{w} + \frac{V_2^2}{2g} = \text{constant} \tag{8}$$

Equation (7) shows that the total energy in each stream tube is the same as in each of the other stream tubes. No energy is

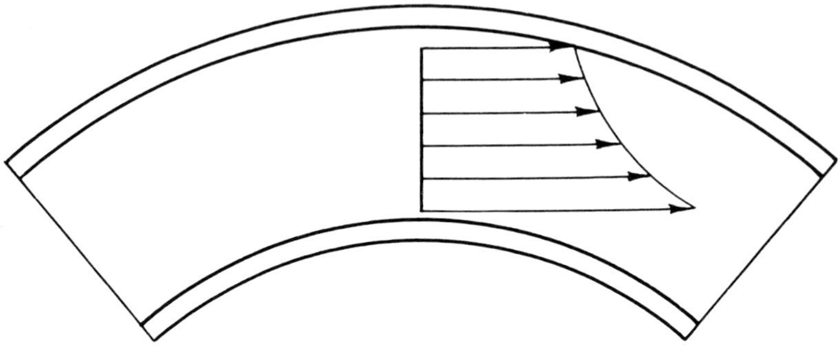

FIGURE 14. Velocity of flow in mainstream at bend. From Texon (1967).

added to the vortex by a torque and no energy is dissipated by friction. Such a free vortex may be found in the two-dimensional flow in the main body of a stream flowing around a bend.

Calculations

In a free vortex the difference in pressure per unit radial distance toward the center is $\rho V^2/r$. Thus, $dp = \rho V^2/r\, dr$. Q (volumetric flow) and A (cross-sectional area) are determined by direct measurement and give V_1 (velocity) because $Q = AV$. When V_1 (velocity) is known and the internal radius of curvature (r_1) and the internal diameter of the vessel (dr) are measured, the difference in pressure on the inner and outer walls of a bend can be calculated from the above equation.

Thus, with a velocity of 25 cm/s and an internal radius of curvature of 1 cm in a vessel having a diameter of 0.3 cm, the difference in pressure is 173 dyn/cm^2, assuming $\rho = 1.06$ g/cm^3 (the density of blood). The radius of curvature of the center line of the vessel is used as the average radius of curvature.

$$
\begin{aligned}
dp &= \rho \left(\frac{V^2}{r}\right) dr \\
V_1 &= 25 \text{ cm/s} \\
r_1 &= 1.15 \text{ cm} \qquad (9) \\
dr &= 0.3 \\
dp &= 173.0 \text{ dyn/cm}^2
\end{aligned}
$$

The difference in pressure *(dp)* will be lessened if the radius of curvature *(r)* is increased or the velocity *(V)* is decreased.

An increase in differential pressure at a bend may be produced by increasing the blood velocity, increasing the diameter (volumetric flow) of the blood vessel at a constant velocity, or by decreasing the radius of curvature. It is known that the potential velocity distribution assumed here will not apply precisely in any actual viscous flow. In actual flow viscous effects cause a portion of the fluid in the region near the wall to be retarded. Outside the wall region the flow may be closer to a free vortex. However, any velocity distribution through the same bend having the same volumetric flow will give the same order of magnitude of pressure differential.

Secondary flow occurs in the flow around a bend in tubes, pipes, and blood vessels. The secondary flow, consisting of two spirals, is superimposed upon the primary or main flow. In rivers and streams the secondary flow tends to pile up sand and gravel at the inner side of the bend and deepen the channel toward the outer side of the bend. No evidence of such deposition of blood elements has been noted in pathological studies of early lesions. Rather it is constantly noted that the diminished lateral pressure on the convex surface of bends stimulates the endothelium to proliferate with production of a progressively thickened intima (see Plate 1) that gradually encroaches upon the lumen as an atherosclerotic plaque. In brief, viscous effects and secondary flow may modify flow in a curved path. These effects may modify the pressure distribution to some extent but cannot eliminate the basic effect of the production of low pressure areas on the convex surface of curved blood vessels that provides the initial stimulus for the development of atherosclerosis.

ATTACHMENT

A free elastic tube has no motion of its wall when the pressures on each side of the wall are equal. The flowing blood, whether steady or oscillating, produces varying pressures that move the wall toward the lesser pressure. Motion of an arterial wall is relatively unrestricted at most points compared to the limitation of motion imposed at zones of attachment (see Figure 9). A localized diminution in lateral pressure at tethered sites occurs during some portion of each heart cycle. It is this mechanical (tensile) stress at points of attachment that stimulates intimal proliferation, the initial change in the development of atherosclerosis.

BRANCHING

Patterns of blood flow at sites of branching are determined by the anatomic pattern of each branch and the rate of flow through each branch. The ratios of branch to parent stem diameter and angles of branching vary greatly. The flow patterns, therefore, necessarily vary and change in accordance with local hydraulic conditions. In the flow pattern of each branch or each bend a zone of relatively low pressure is produced (Figures 12 and 15). If a sufficient suction effect due to the diminished lateral pressure is produced, an intimal response leading to atherosclerosis may appear.

Ostial Lesions

Ostial lesion is the term applied to the intimal changes, including atherosclerotic plaques, that occur at the zone of origin of a branch vessel. These lesions are here interpreted as the local biologic response of the blood vessel to the hydraulic forces generated by the flowing blood. Although the patterns of flow at a branch necessarily vary because of variations in pulsatile flow as well as variations in geometry or anatomical design, idealized situations may be analyzed precisely and may serve as basis for interpreting more complex patterns of flow. The distribution of the pathological changes (Bjorkerus and Bondjers, 1972) reflects the predominant pattern of flow as well as the change in pattern of flow due to the progressively developing anatomical lesion itself. The atherosclerotic plaque is, in effect, the composite result of all the pertinent hydraulic conditions. These may include pulse rate, stroke volume, rhythm, amplitude, elasticity, ratio of the diameter of the main stem to branch diameter, shape of the ostial orifice, angle of branching, and velocity of flow.

The laws of fluid mechanics determine that the pattern of flow at the site of a branch is usually characterized by several zones of diminished lateral pressure. These may be identified at points D_1 and D_2 (Figure 15). The relatively high shear stress at point F reflects the increased velocity gradient adjacent to the wall surface or at the interface.

It is notable that in any branching anatomical pattern a stagnation point must develop at the distal margin of the ostial orifice. The stagnation point is a point of high pressure and

COLOR PLATE LEGENDS

PLATE 1. Dog no. 5311, femoral artery: (A) normal endothelial layer with subjacent internal elastic membrane; (B, C) progressive intimal thickening with normal internal elastic membrane.

PLATE 2. (A) White woman, age 23, aorta—intimal proliferation with lipid changes in basement zone of the atherosclerotic plaque. Note orientation of nuclci in direction of blood flow. (B) White man, age 54, aortic intimal proliferation with lipid in basement zone of plaque. (C) Dog no. 1271 A (normal diet), coronary artery—left anterior descending branch showing early lipid change, droplets within fibroblasts in basement zone of intimal plaque.

PLATE 3. Dog no. 2134, carotid artery—hemorrhage within atherosclerotic plaque. From Texon (1967).

PLATE 4. White woman, age 29, coronary artery (L.A.D.)—advanced atherosclerosis with almost complete occlusion of lumen. From Texon (1974).

PLATE 5. Human, ostial lesions—atherosclerotic plaques in dorsal aorta distal to origin of intercoastal arteries—the localized biological response to the local pattern of blood flow that produces the localized low pressure zone. Note the linear atherosclerotic plaques on the posterior wall (attachment lesions). From Texon (1972).

PLATE 6. (A, B) Dog, cross sections normal to axis of femoral artery. Typical ostial lesions are observed at the junction of the parent vessel with a branch. These lesions may also be associated with a separated flow that occurs early in systole when velocity of flow in the parent vessel is first increasing rapidly. From Texon (1972).

PLATE 7. Bifurcation of the aorta showing "crotch," "bifurcation," or "Y" lesions of the common iliac arteries. Note intramural hemorrhage. From Texon (1963).

PLATE 8. (A, B, C) Bifurcation of the human aorta—three autopsy specimens *in situ*. Note variation in the internal angle of bifurcation: (A) = 40°, (B) = 45°, (C) = 50°. From Texon (1976a).

PLATE 9. Black woman, age 62: (A) bifurcation of the aorta. Note relatively acute internal angle (26°); (B) medial walls of the iliac arteries showing atherosclerosis. From Texon (1976a).

PLATE 10. White woman, age 15, coronary atherosclerosis–linear atherosclerotic plaques in curvature lesions: (A) left anterior descending branch; (B) right coronary artery. From Texon (1976b).

PLATE 11. Atherosclerotic plaque on inner (convex) wall of aortic arch, opposite origins of great vessels. Note dorsal wall "attachment" lesion in thoracic aorta.

PLATE 12. Thoracic aorta. Note "attachment" lesions on dorsal wall. Note also the "ostial" lesions. From Texon (1963).

PLATE 13. Atherosclerotic plaque with ulceration on medial wall of iliac artery. Note that proximal margin of the plaque is about 1 cm distal to the carina or margin of the bifurcation. From Texon (1976a).

PLATE 14. Splenic artery. Note the atherosclerotic plaque on the convex surface of each of three curvatures. From Texon (1963).

PLATE 15. White woman, age 23, ostial lesions in aorta, distal to orifices of intercostal arteries.

PLATE 16. (A, B) Dog no. 5278, femoral artery–intimal proliferation at zone of tensile stress in a branch normal to direction of main flow.

PLATE 17. White woman, age 54, ductus arteriosus–gross specimen. From Texon (1974).

PLATE 18. Ductus arteriosus–obliteration of lumen by occlusive fibroblastic proliferation. From Texon (1974).

PLATE 19. Ductus arteriosus (H.P.)–microscopic–showing remnants of internal elastic membrane in the lumen obliterated by fibroblastic proliferation. From Texon (1974).

PLATE 20. White female, age 6 months: (A) coronary artery (L.A.D.); (B) detail of left edge of artery (A), showing normal intima; (C) detail of right edge of artery (A), showing intimal thickening in a "curvature" lesion. From Texon (1976).

PLATE 21. Dog no. 2211. Curvature preparation–femoral artery autografted to transected carotid artery–pathological changes at zones of curvatures, tapering, and external attachment. Dates of surgery, 11/3/61–12/6/63 (25 months)–normal diet: (A) surgical preparation–curvatures–11/3/63; (B) carotid artery with normal intima; (C) normal intima (endothelial layer) and normal internal elastic layer; (D) eccentric intimal proliferation; (E) concentric intimal proliferation; (F) intimal proliferation (medium power); (G) concentric intimal proliferation with tongue-like projection into lumen; (H) concentric intimal proliferation with further tongue-like projection and encroachment upon the lumen; (I) eccentric intimal proliferation with more than 50% occlusion of lumen; (J) intimal proliferation with degenerative changes in the eccentric plaque; (K) eccentric intimal plaque with markedly diminished lumen; (L) occlusive intimal proliferation with residual lumina.

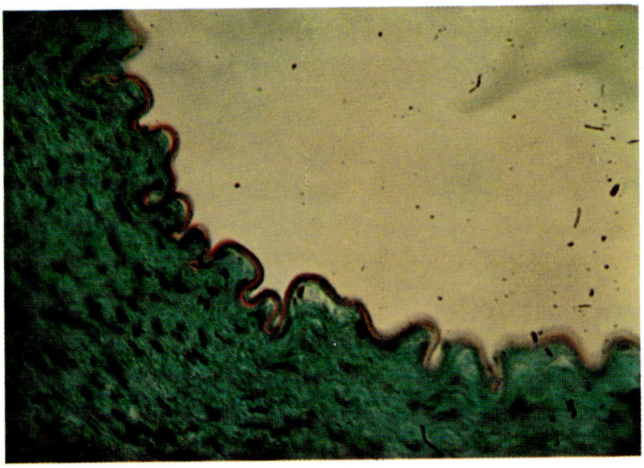

PLATE 1A

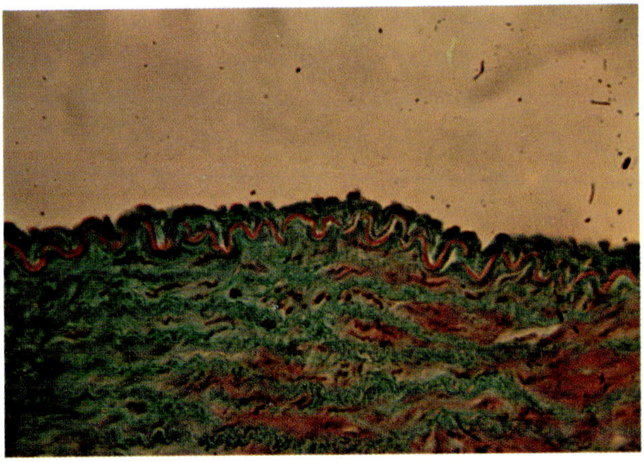

PLATE 1B

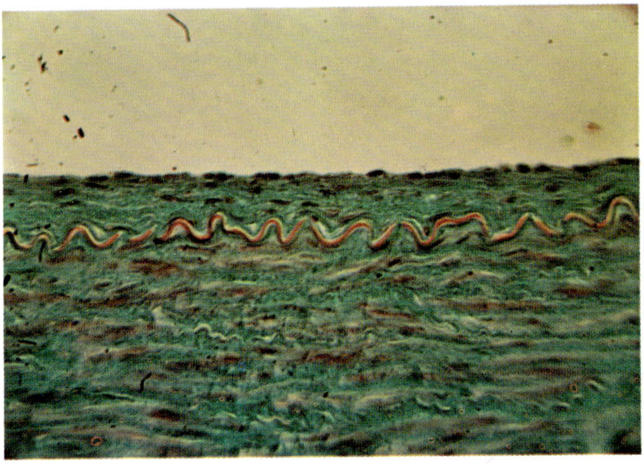

PLATE 1C

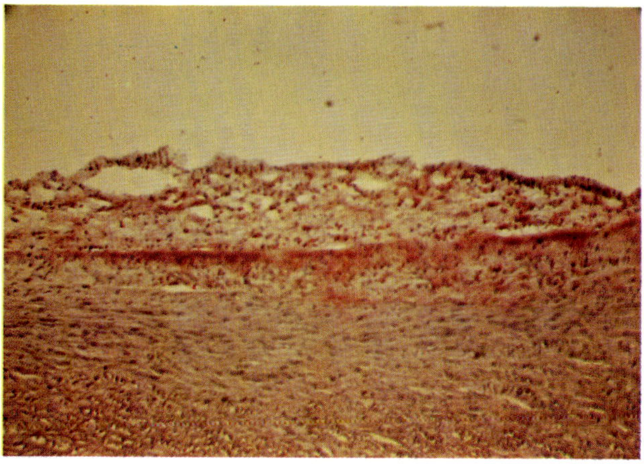

PLATE 2A

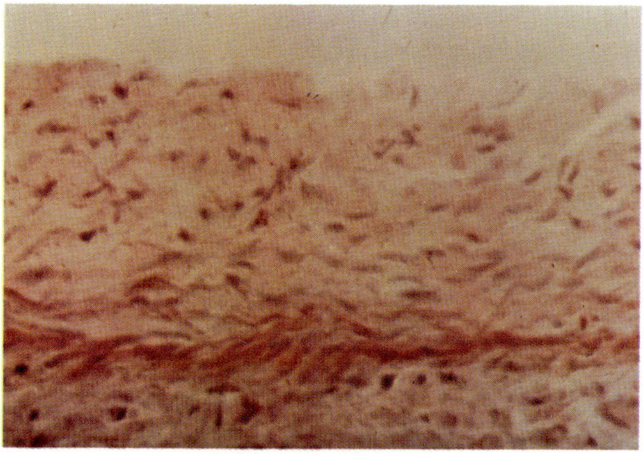

PLATE 2B

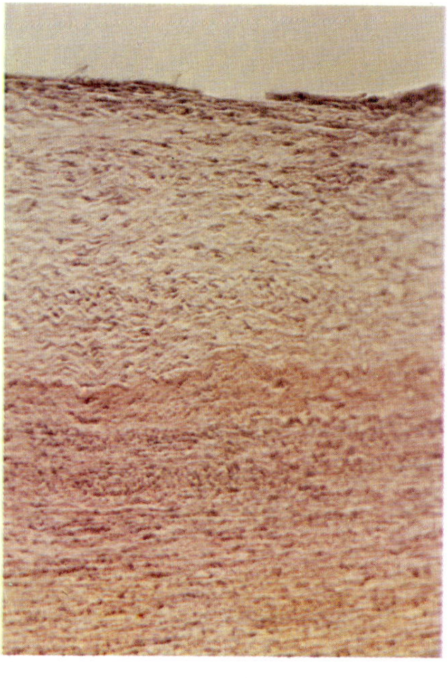

PLATE 2C

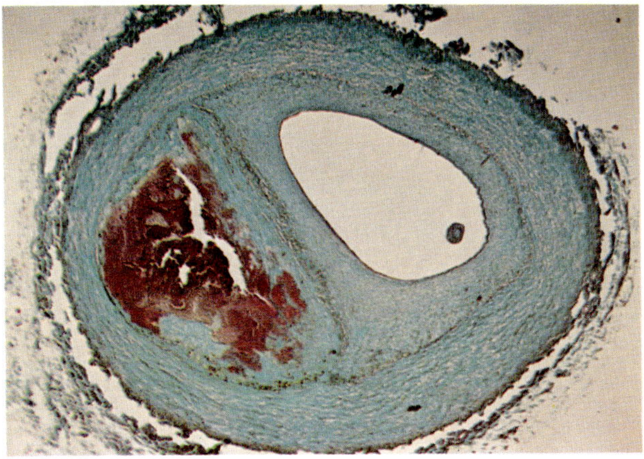

PLATE 3

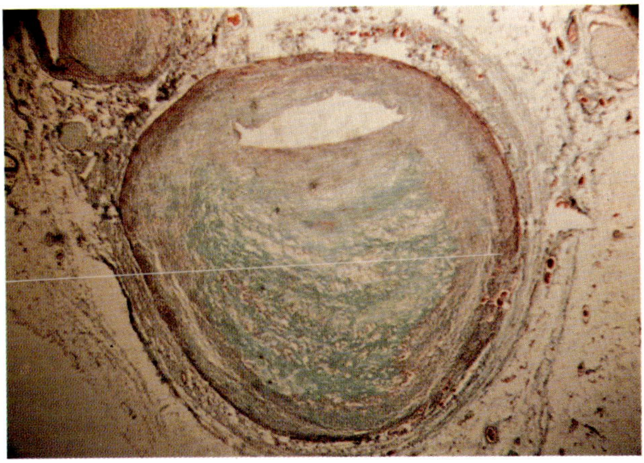

PLATE 4

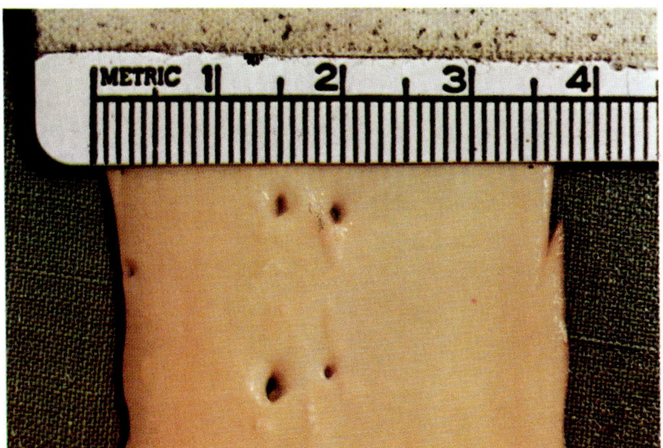

PLATE 5

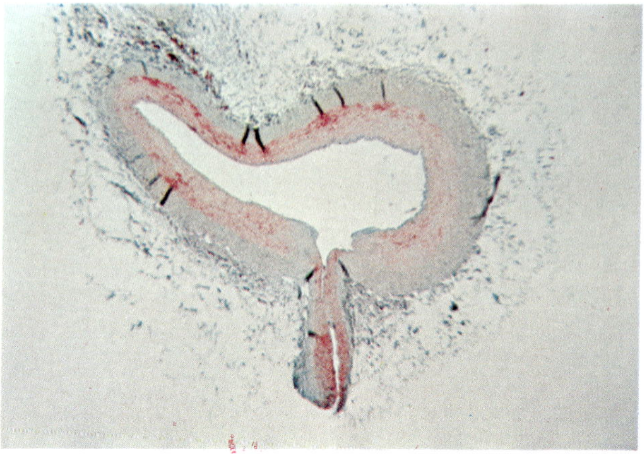

PLATE 6A

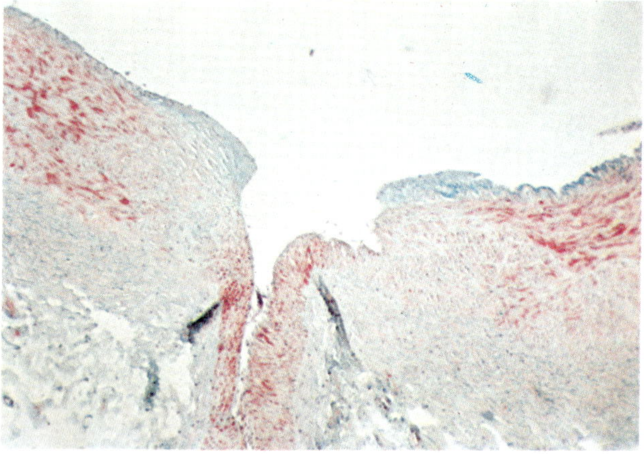

PLATE 6B

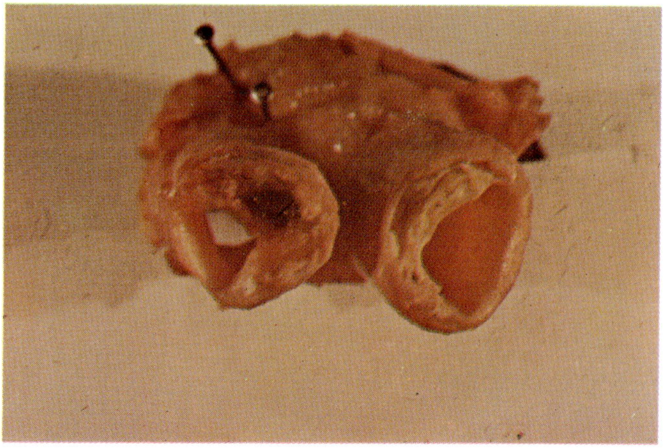

PLATE 7

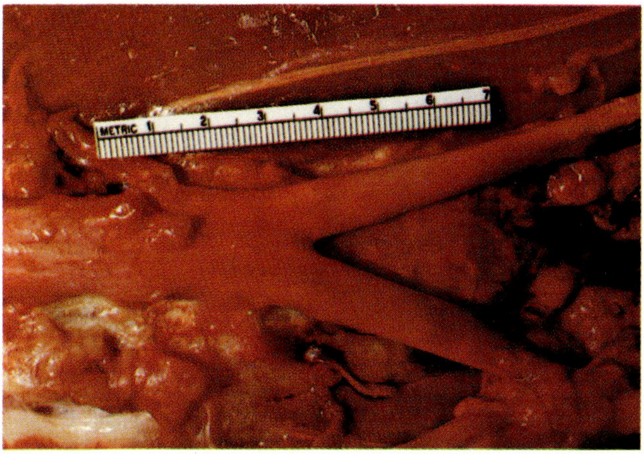

PLATE 8A

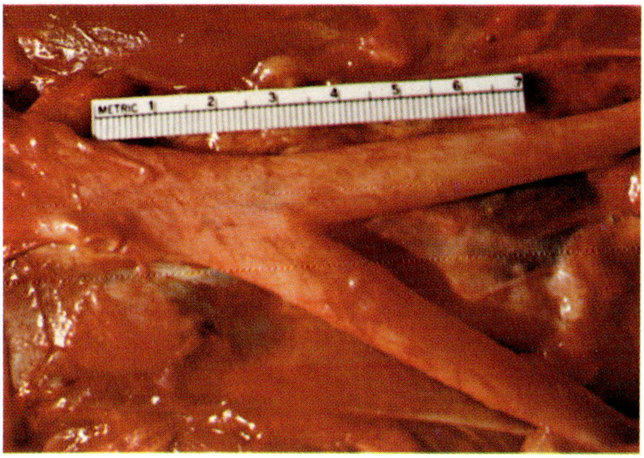

PLATE 8B

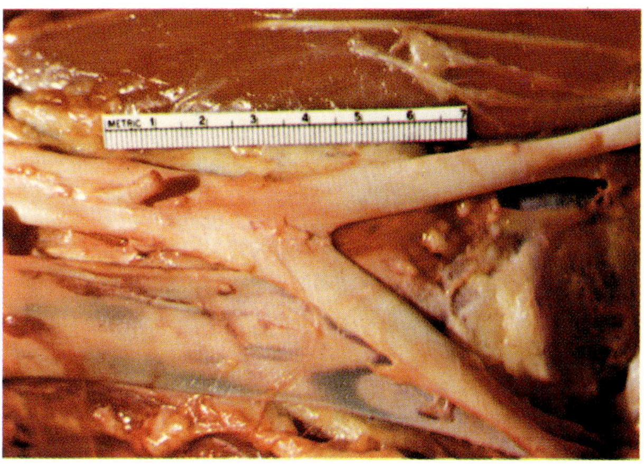

PLATE 8C

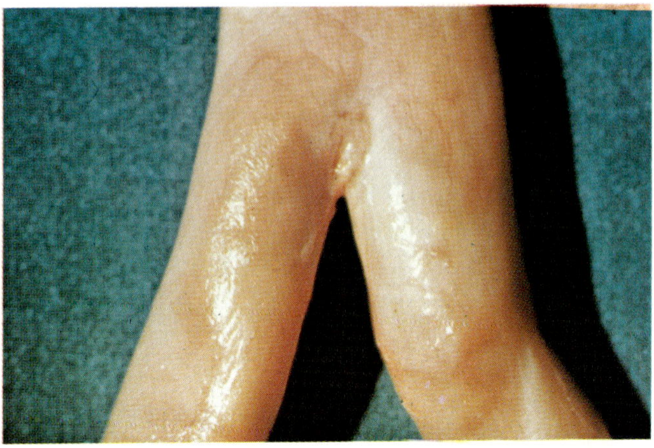

PLAT

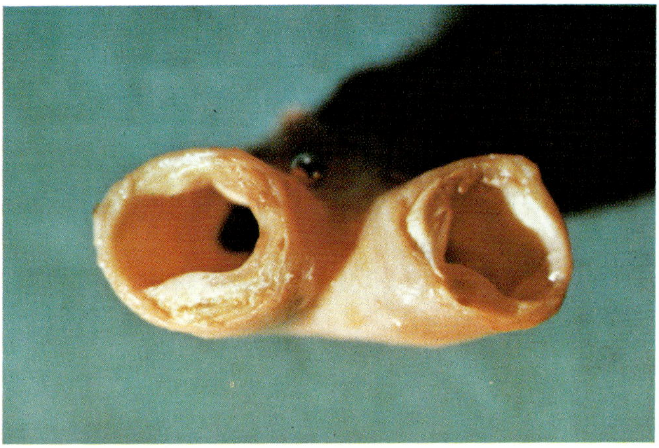

PLAT

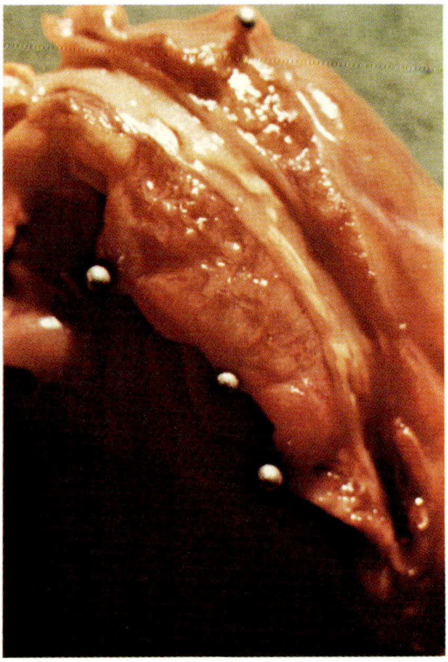

PLATE 10A

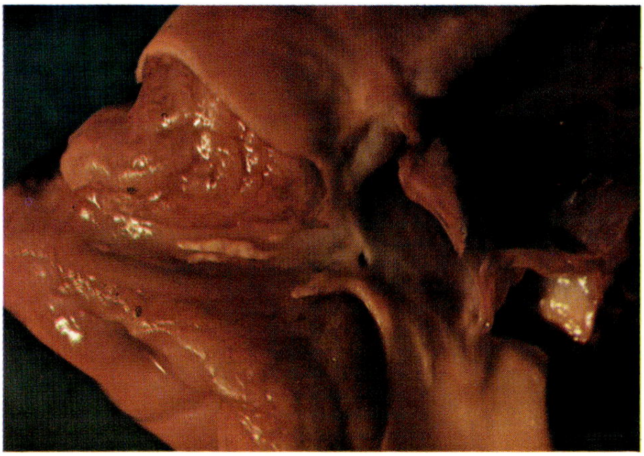

PLATE 10B

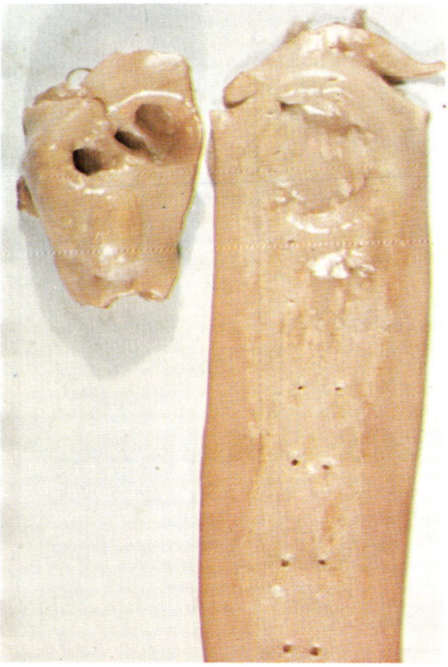

PLATE 11

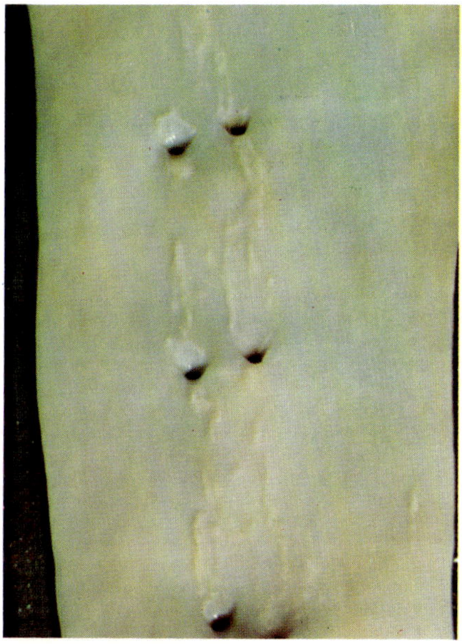

PLATE 12

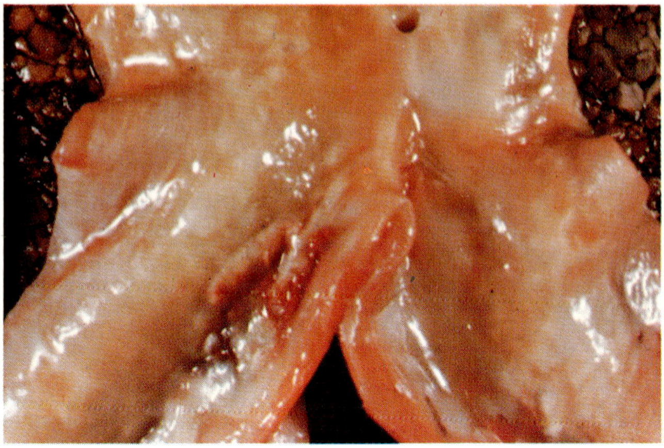

PLATE 13

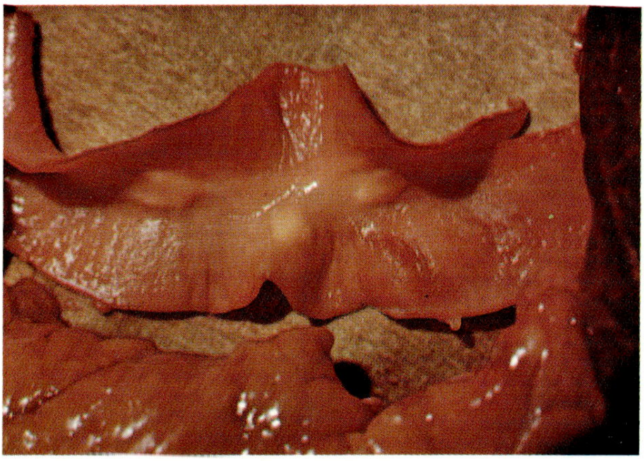

PLATE 14

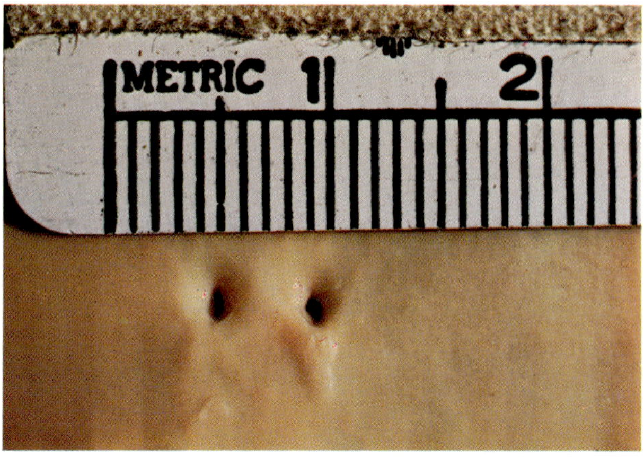

PLATE 15

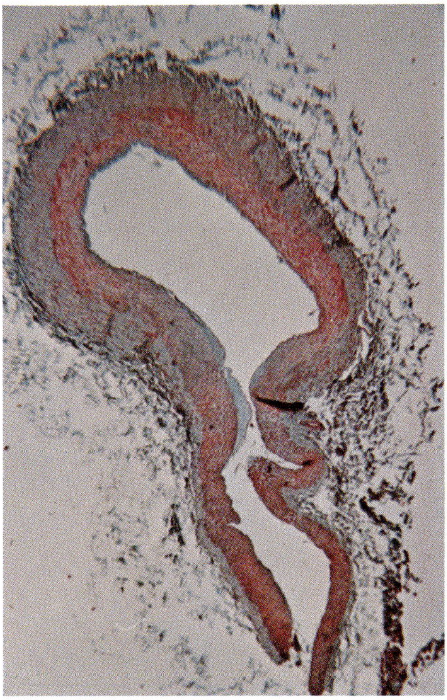

PLATE 16A

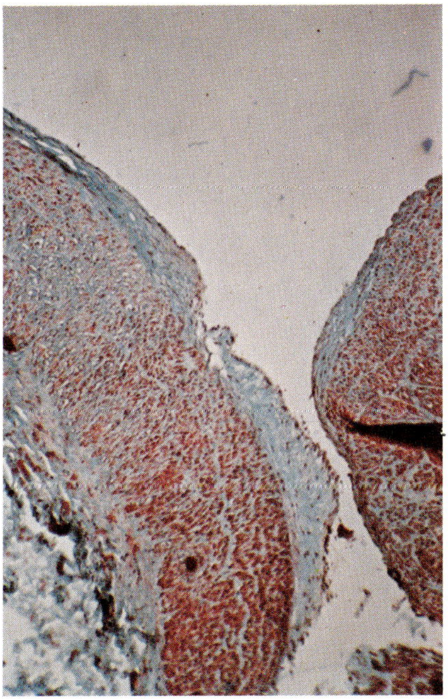

PLATE 16B

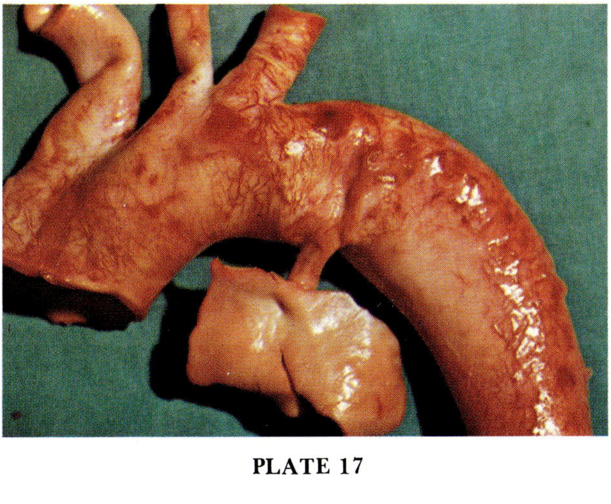

PLATE 17

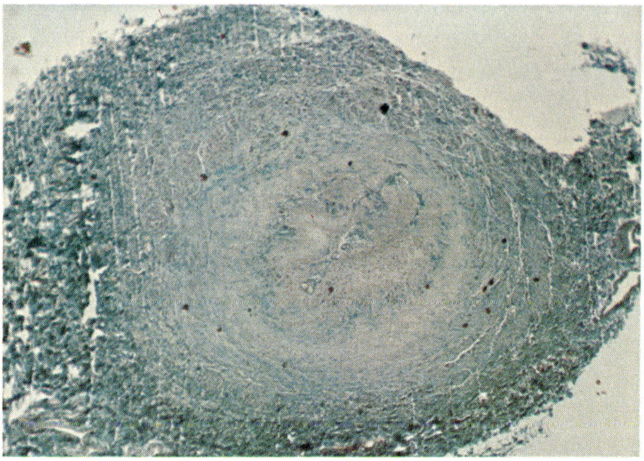

PLATE 18

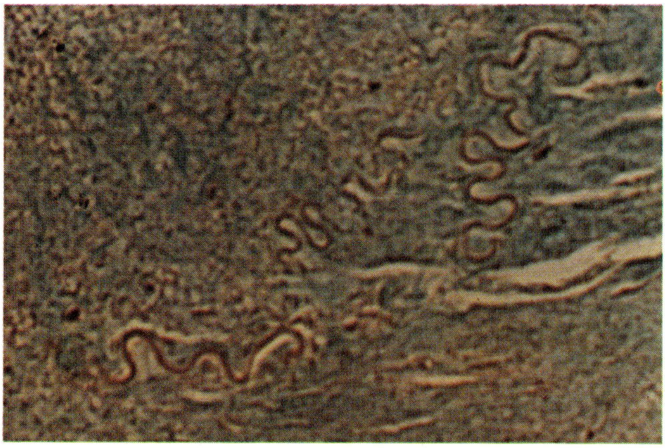

PLATE 19

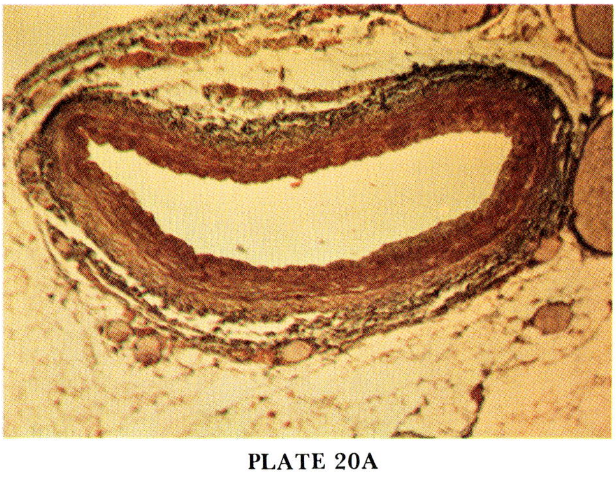

PLATE 20A

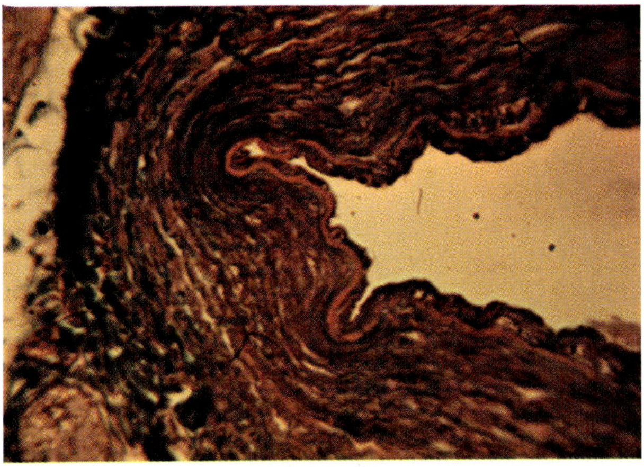

PLATE 20B

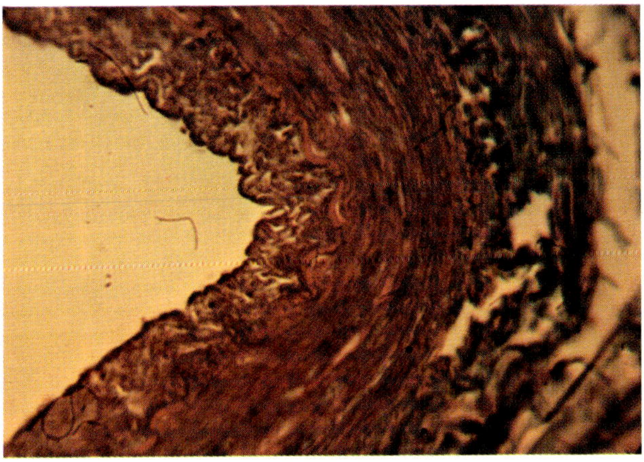

PLATE 20C

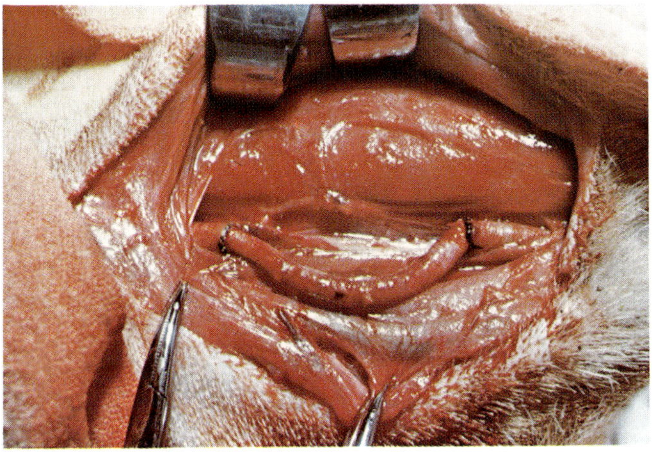

PLATE 21A

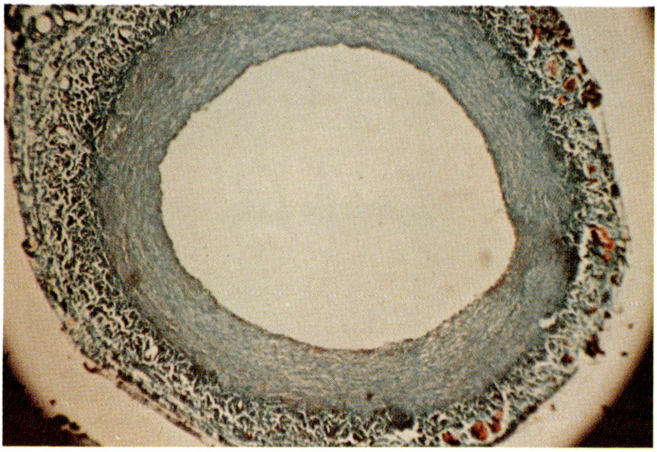

PLATE 21B

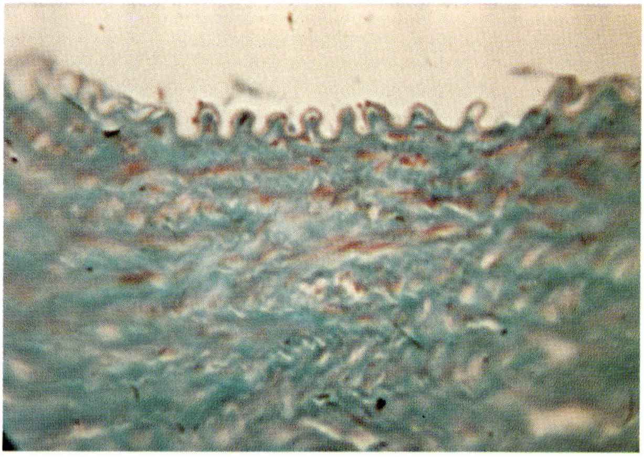

PLATE 21C

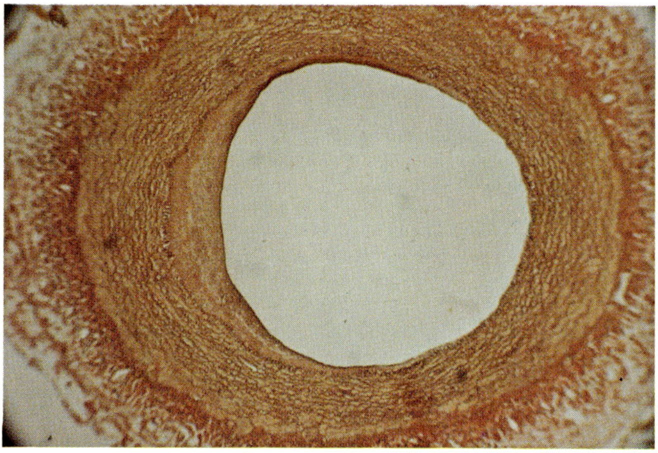

PLATE 21D

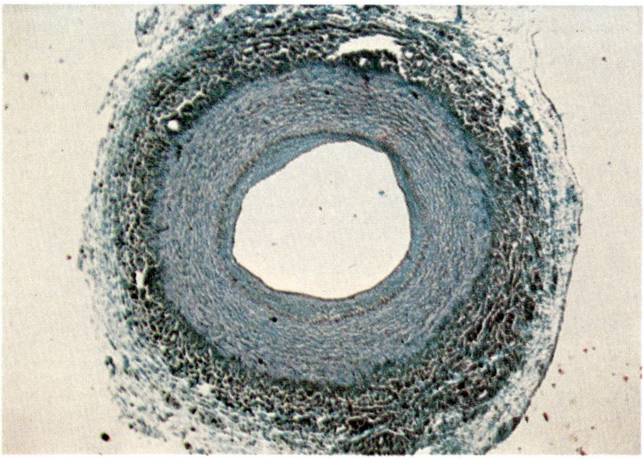

PLATE 21E

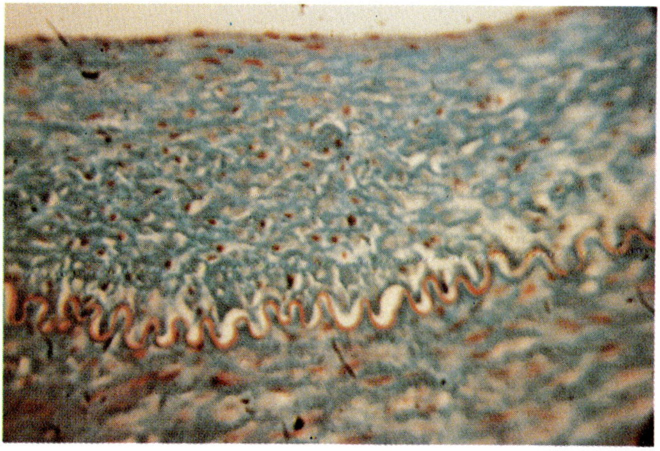

PLATE 21F

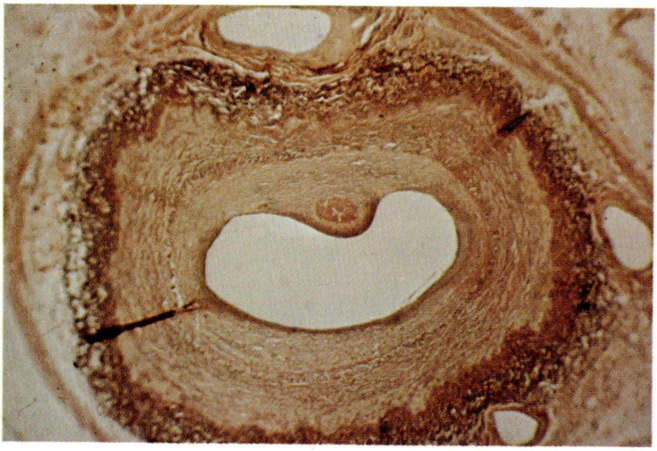

PLATE 21G

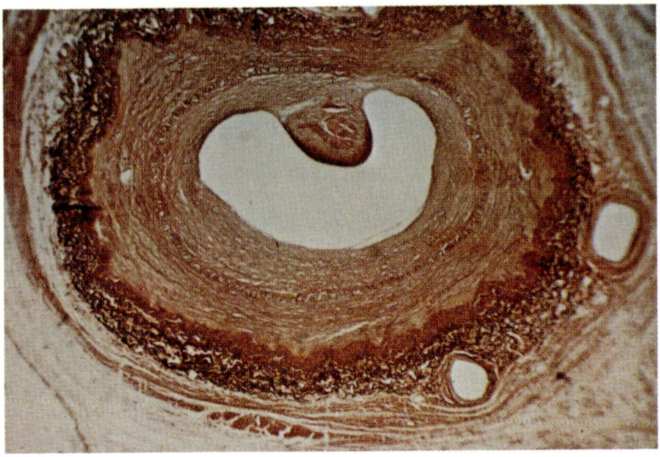
PLATE 21H

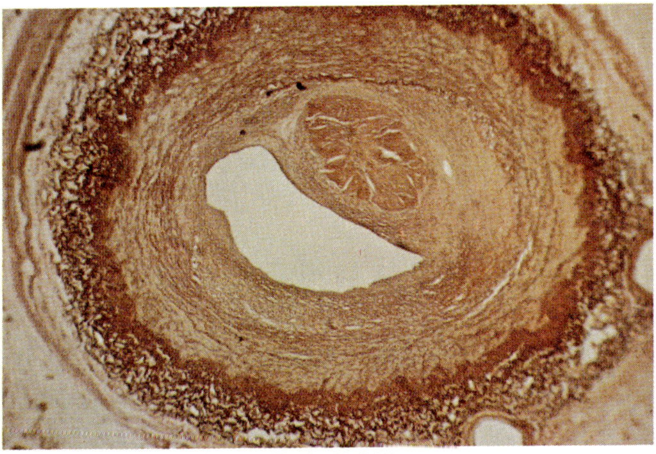
PLATE 21I

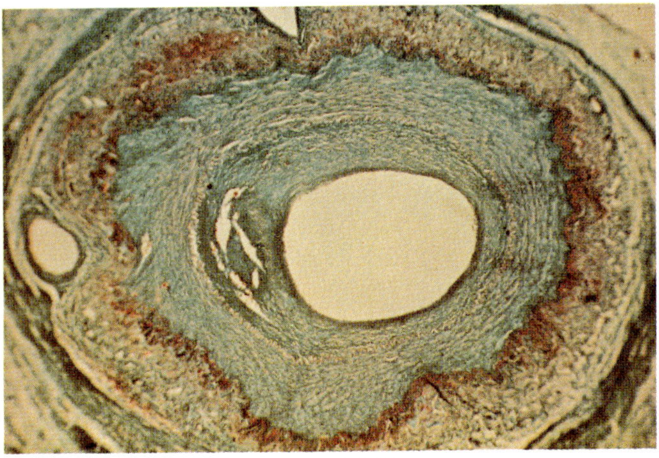
PLATE 21J

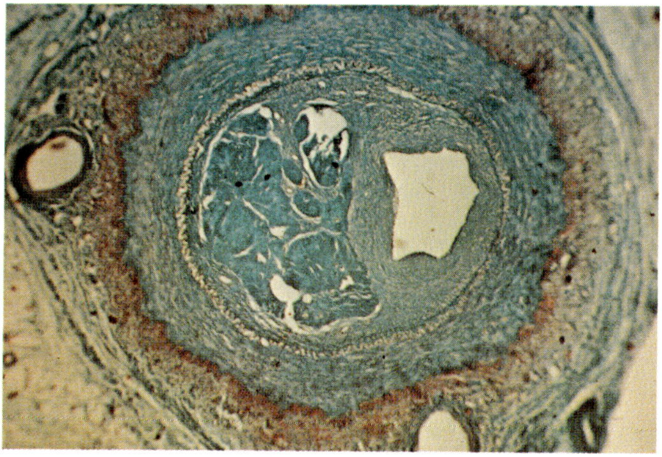

PLATE 21K

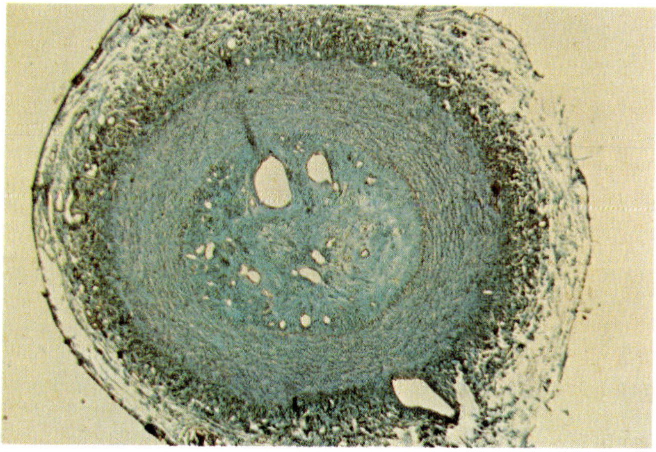

PLATE 21L

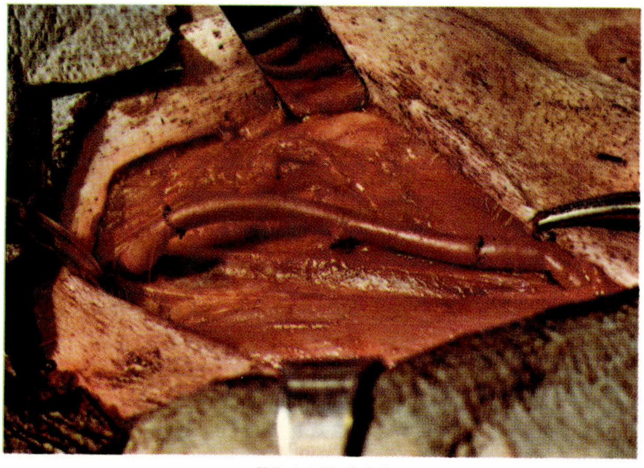

PLATE 22A

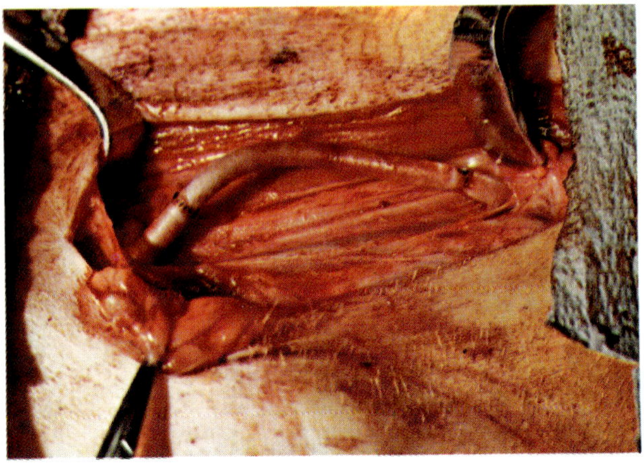

PLATE 22B

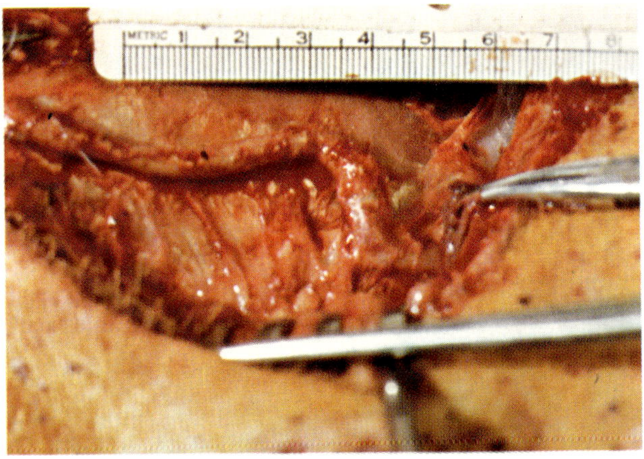

PLATE 22C

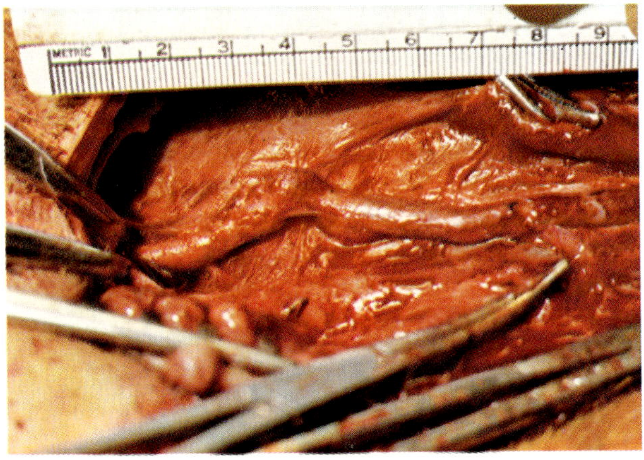

PLATE 22D

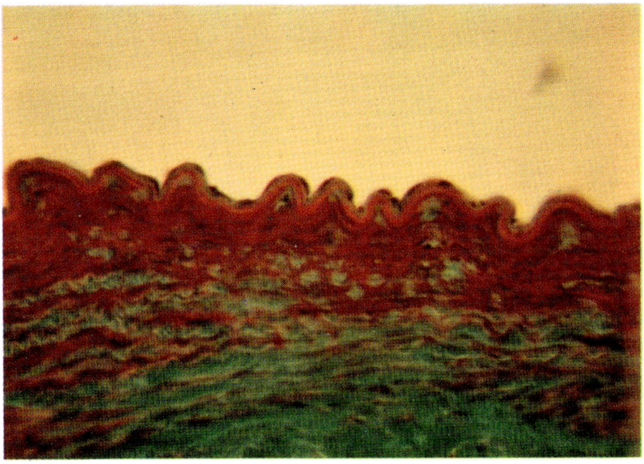

PLATE 22E

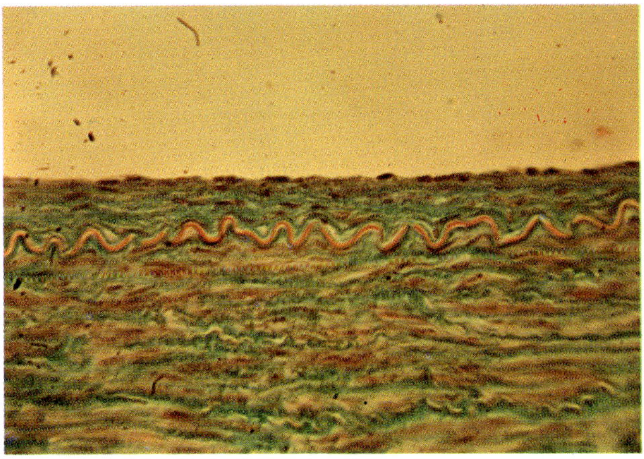

PLATE 22F

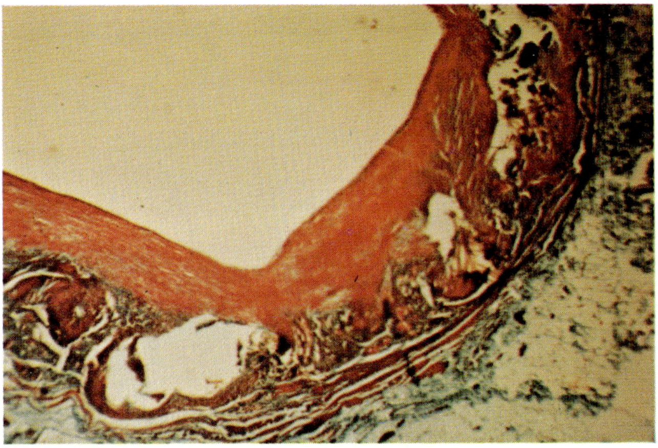

PLATE 22G

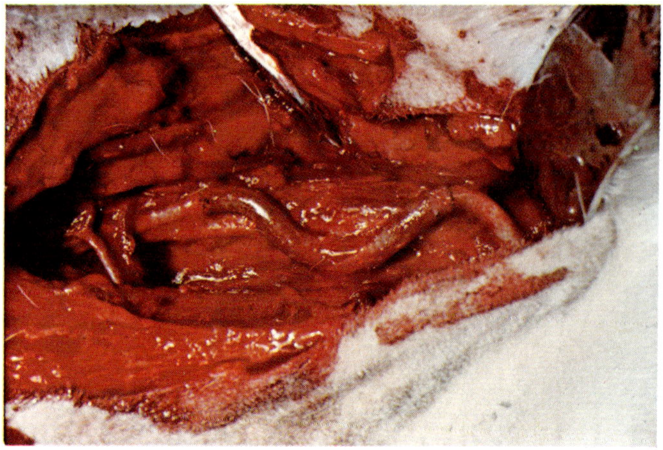

PLATE 23A

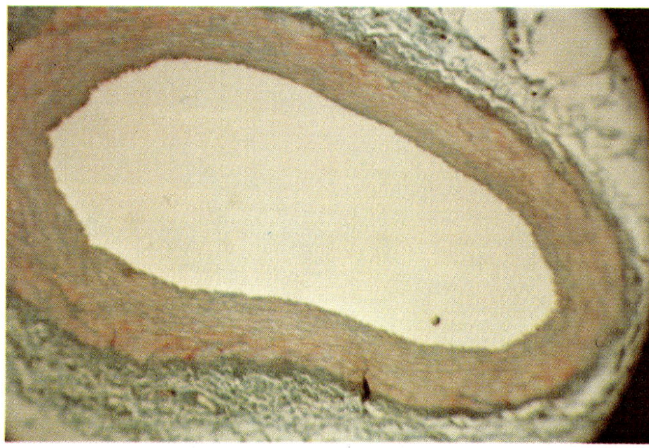

PLATE 23B

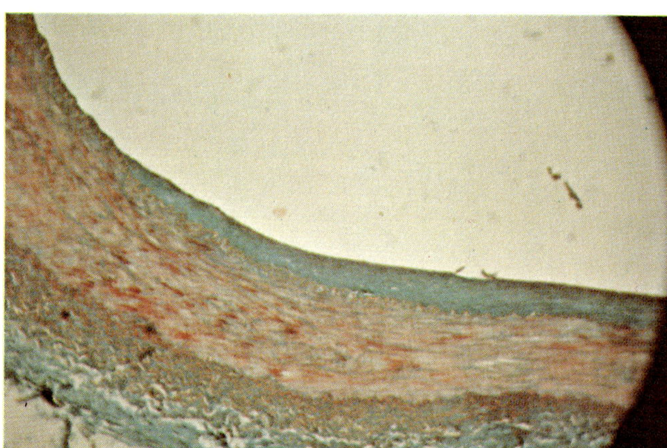

PLATE 23C

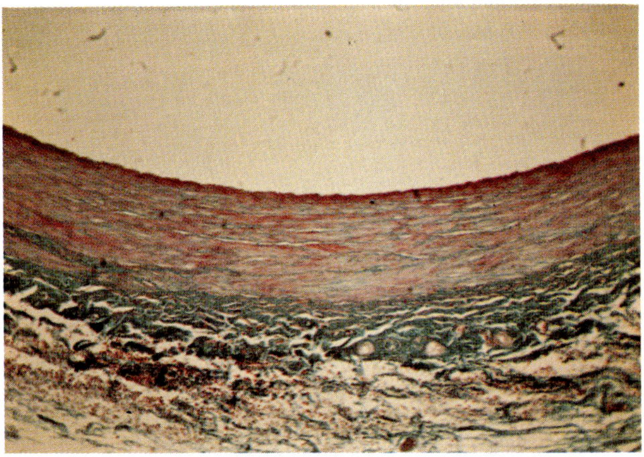

PLATE 23D

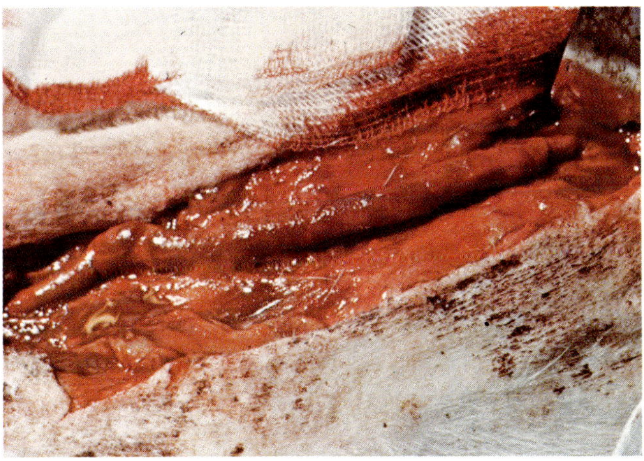

PLATE 23E

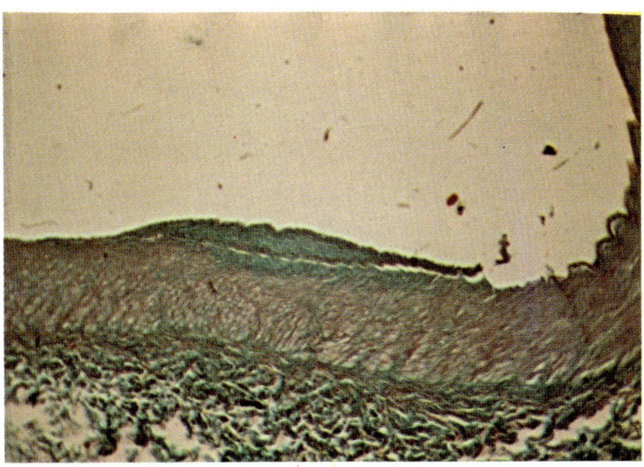

PLATE 23F

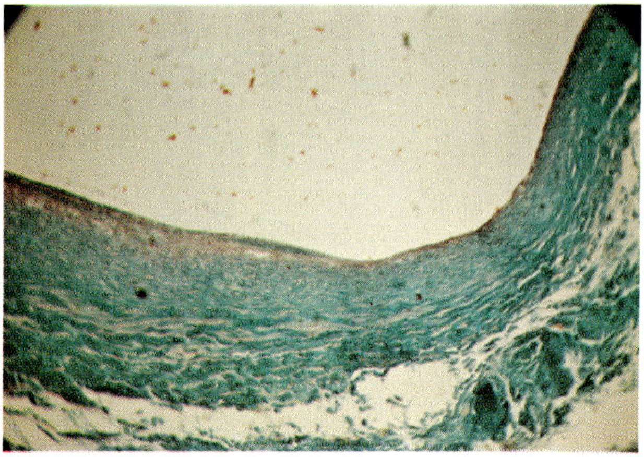

PLATE 23G

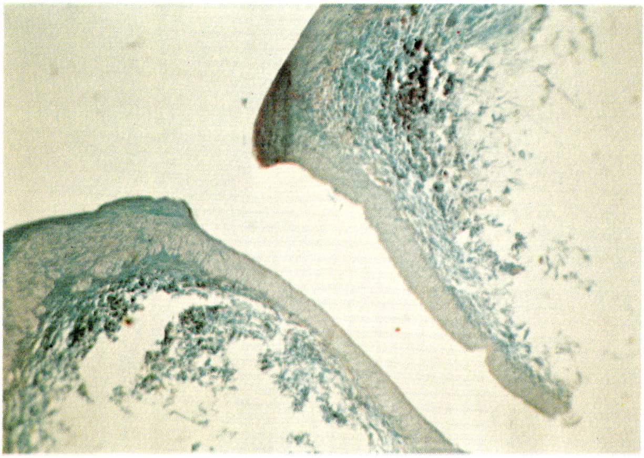

PLATE 23H

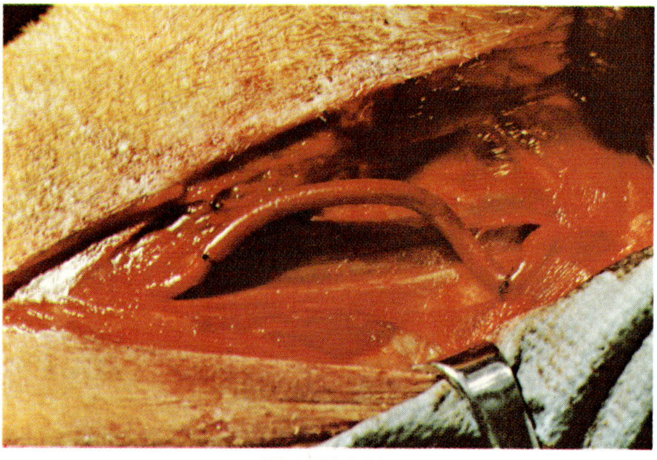

PLATE 24A

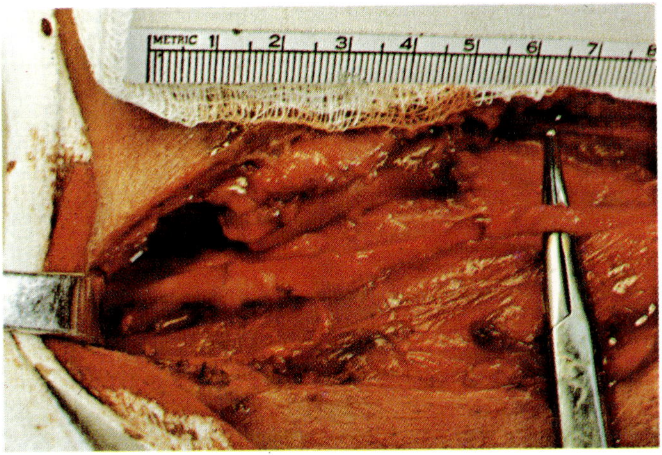

PLATE 24B

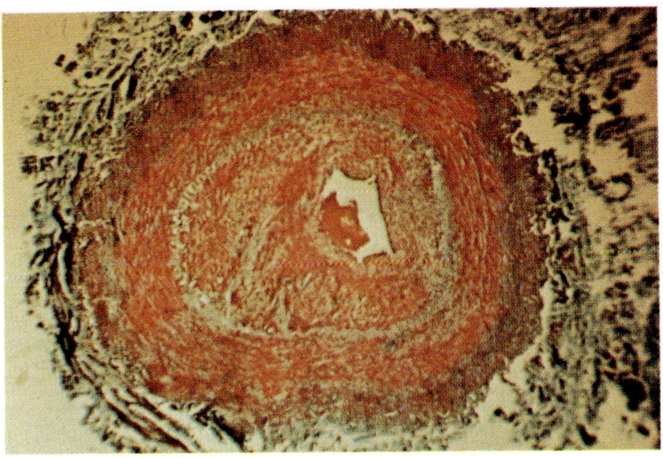

PLATE 24C

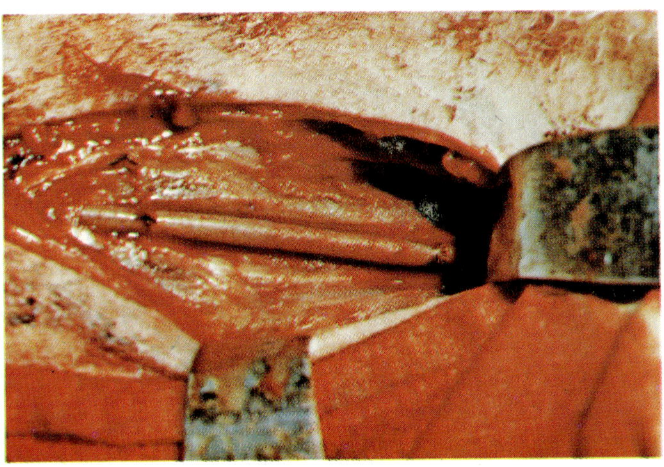

PLATE 25A

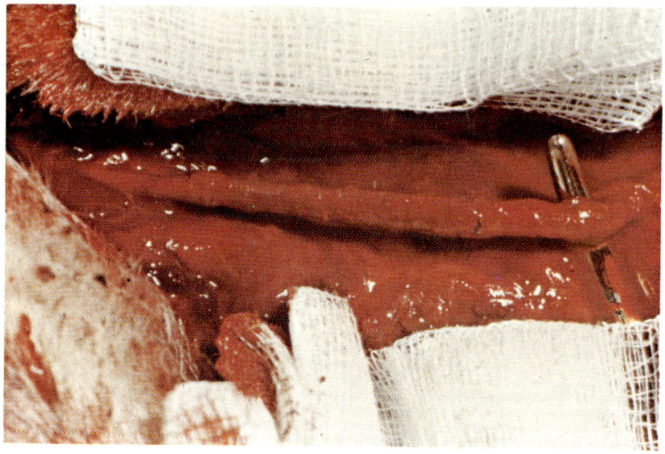

PLATE 25B

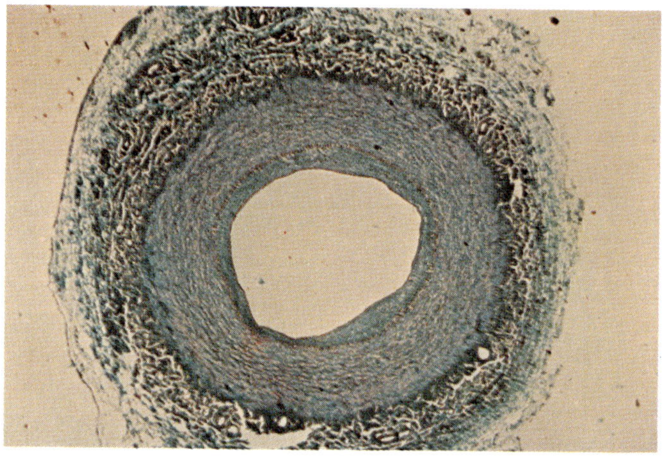

PLATE 25C

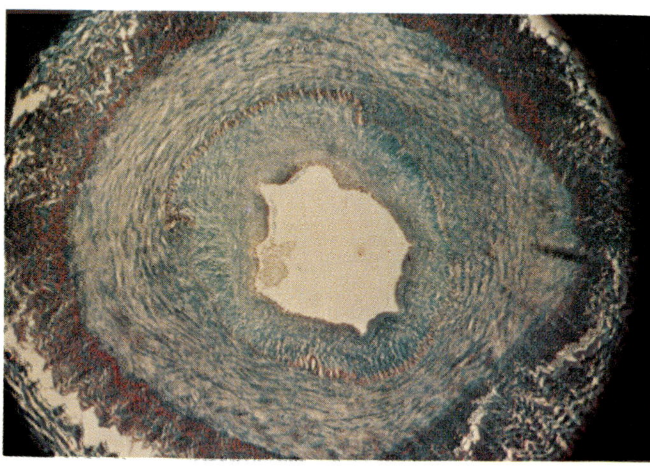

PLATE 25D

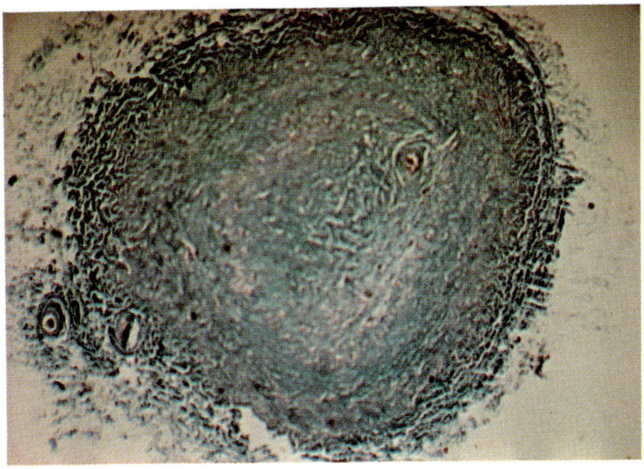

PLATE 25E

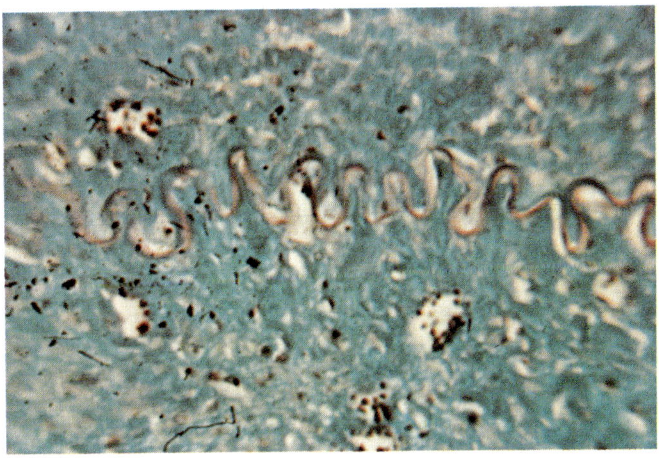

PLATE 25F

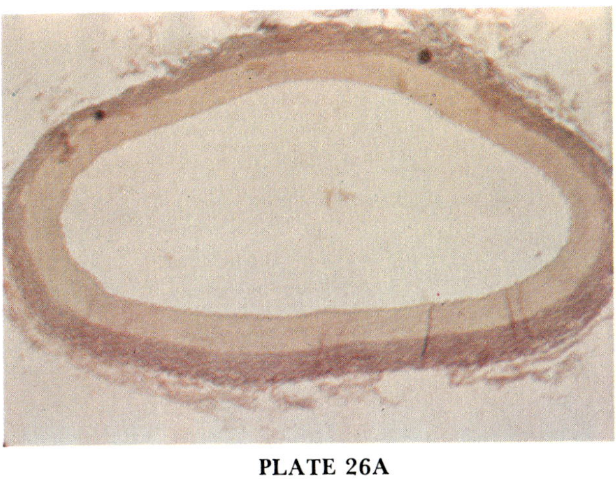

PLATE 26A

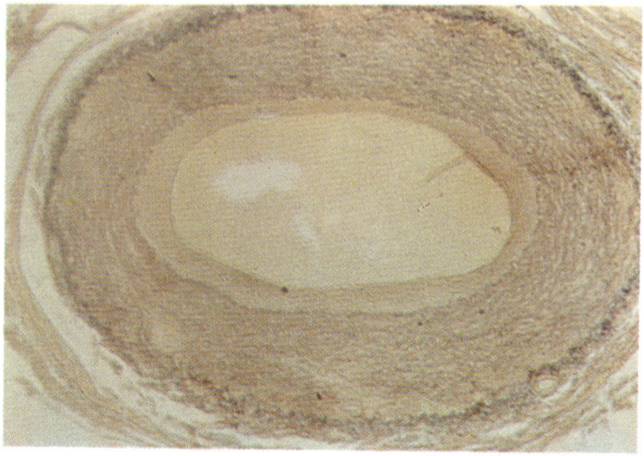

PLATE 26B

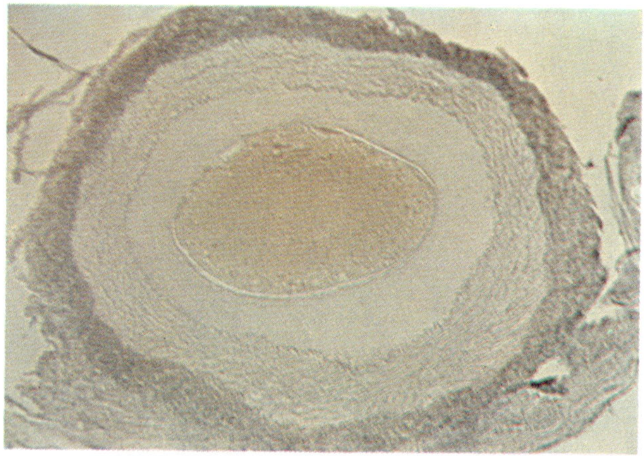

PLATE 26C

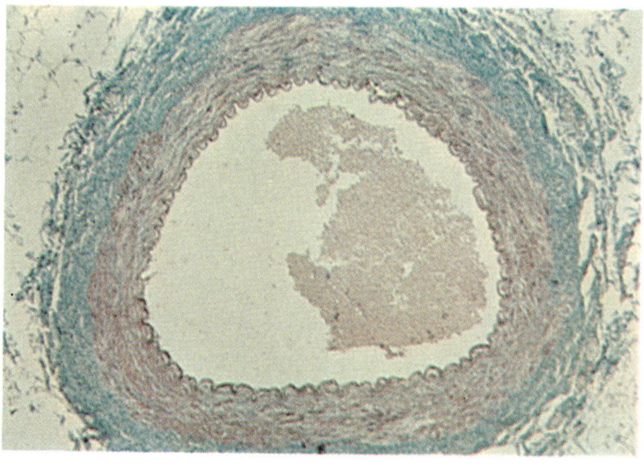

PLATE 26D

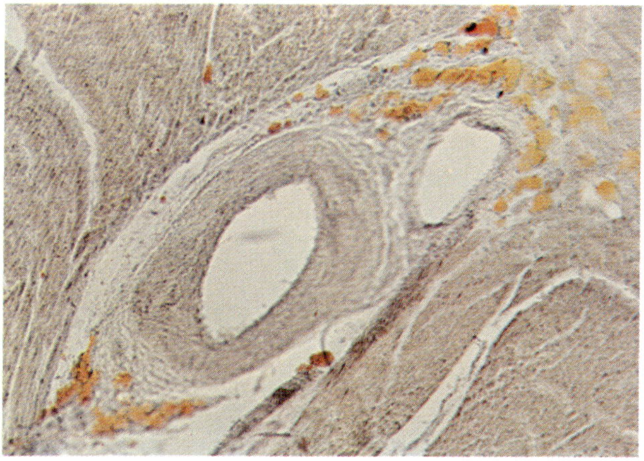

PLATE 26E

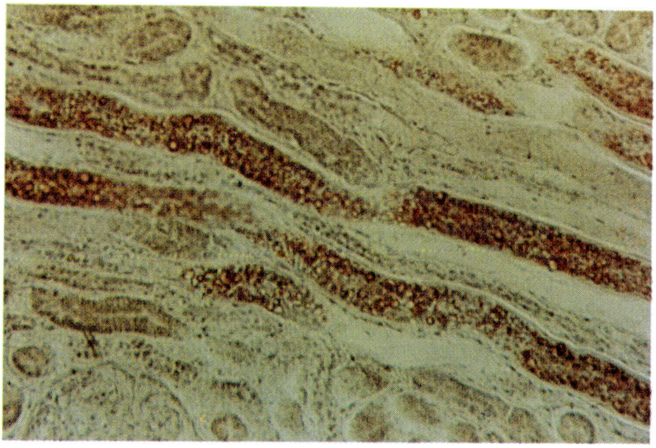

PLATE 26F

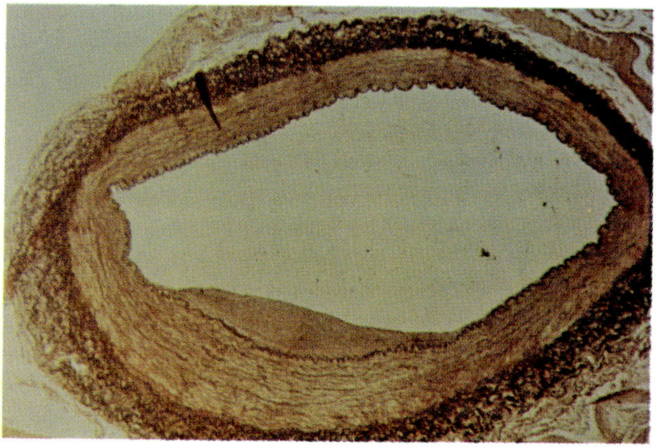

PLATE 27A

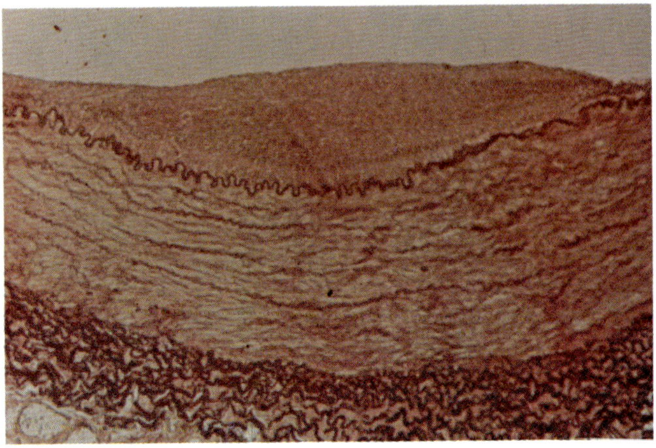

PLATE 27B

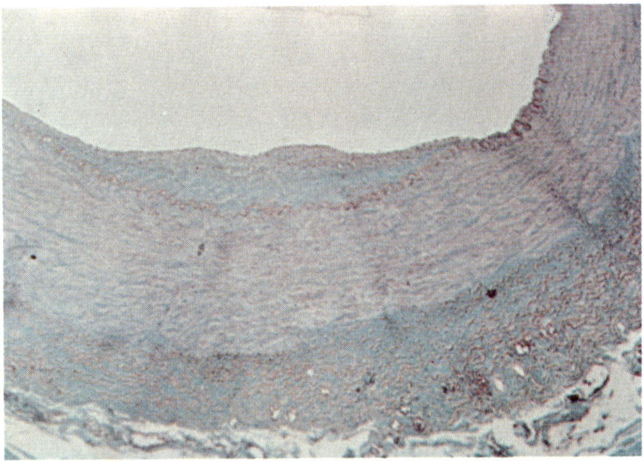

PLATE 27C

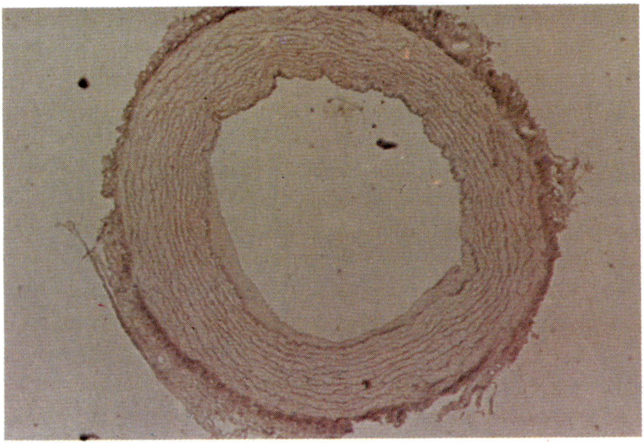

PLATE 27D

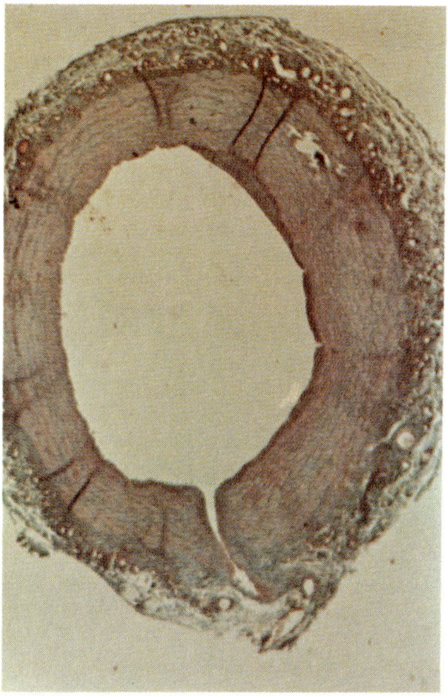

PLATE 27E

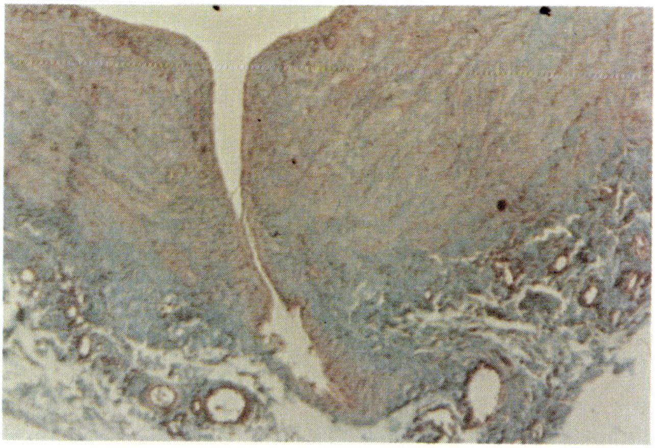

PLATE 27F

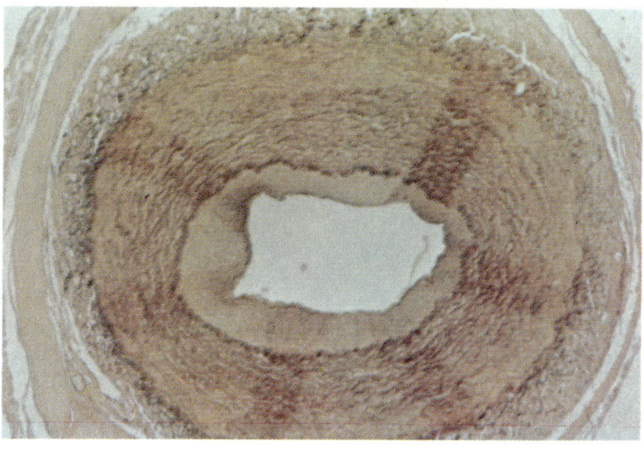

PLATE 28A

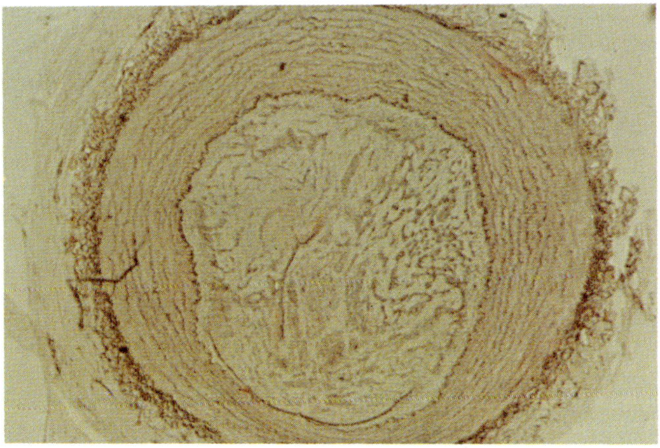

PLATE 28B

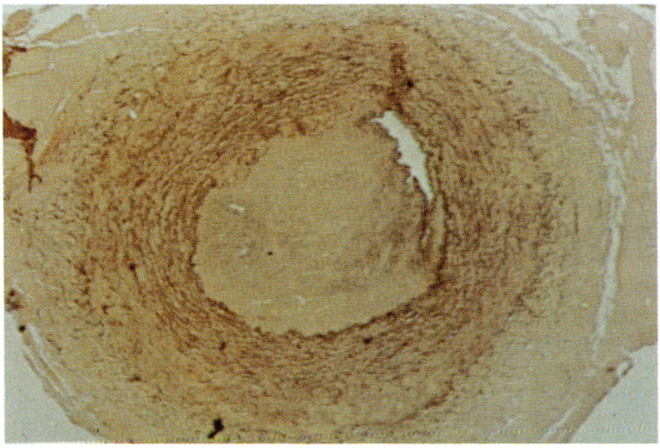

PLATE 28C

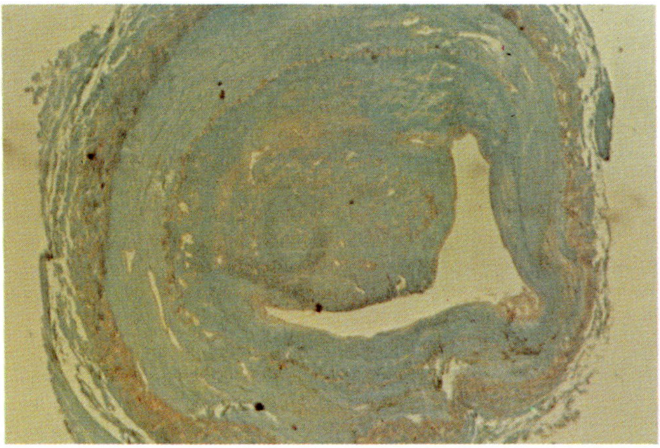

PLATE 28D

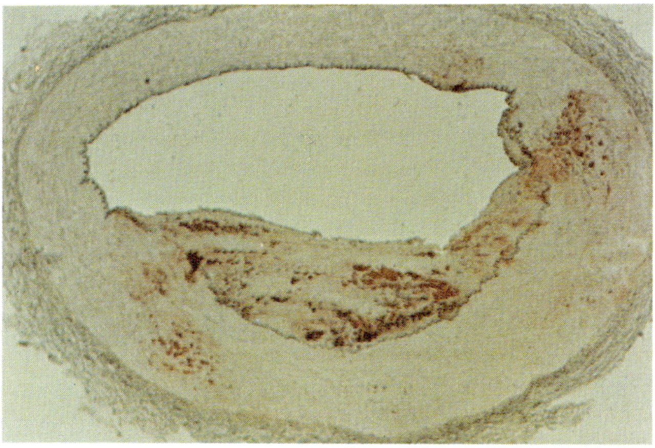

PLATE 28E

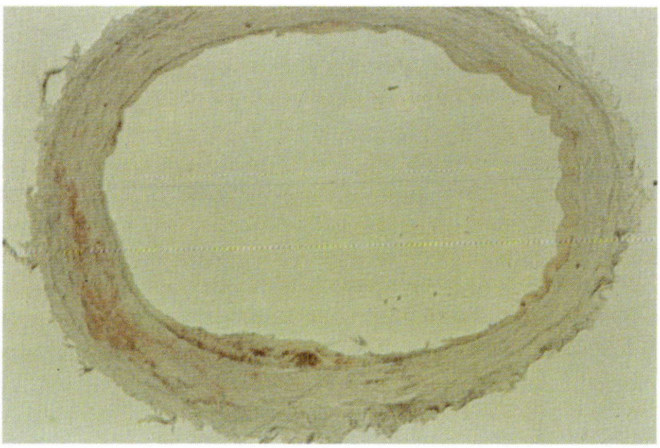

PLATE 28F

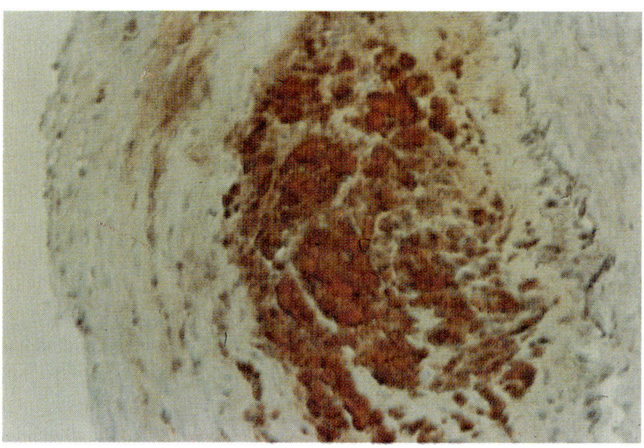

PLATE 28G

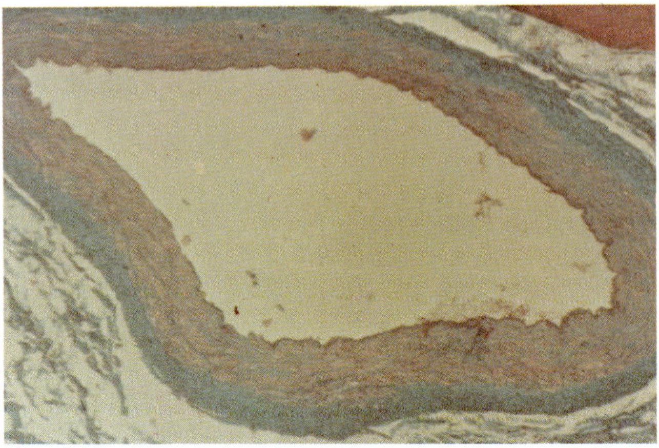

PLATE 28H

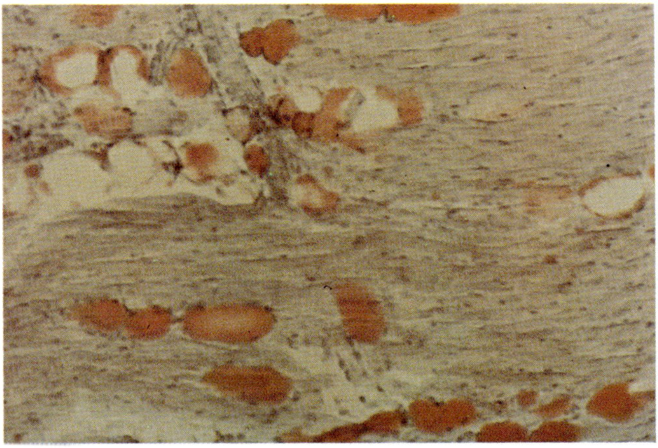

PLATE 28I

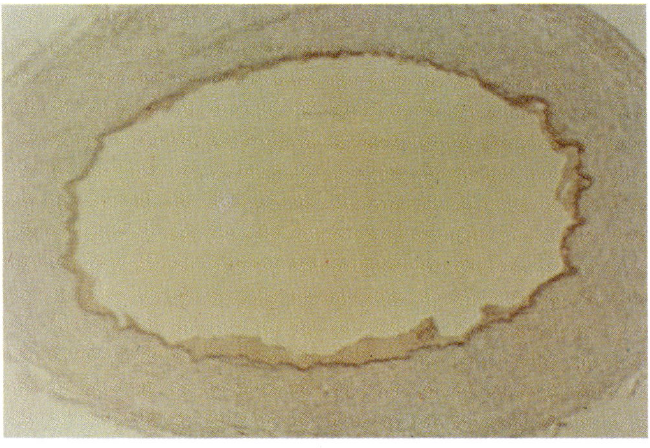

PLATE 28J

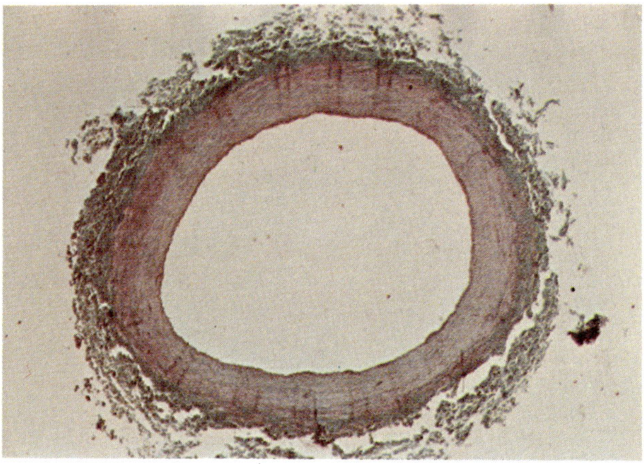

PLATE 29A

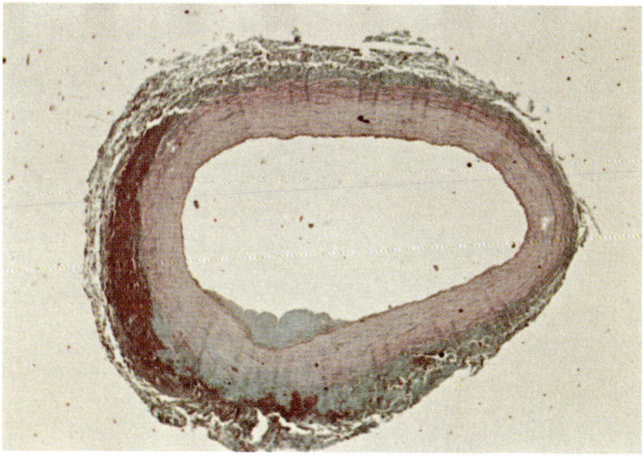

PLATE 29B

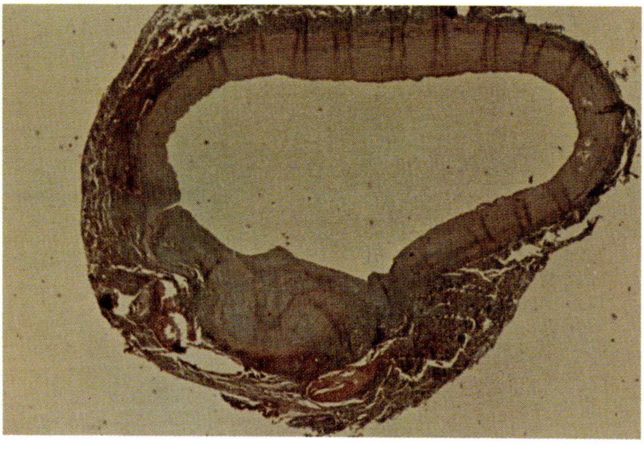

PLATE 29C

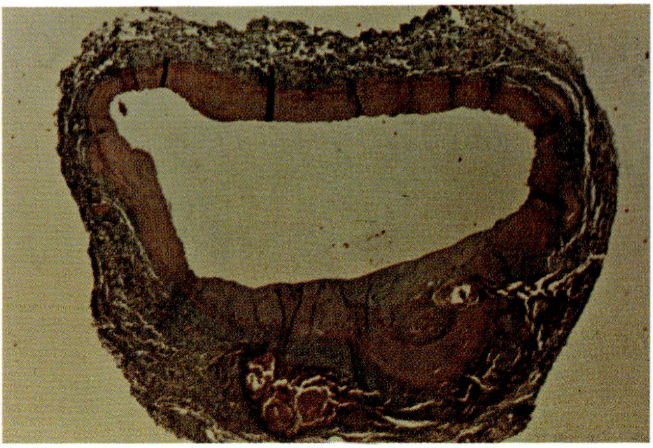

PLATE 29D

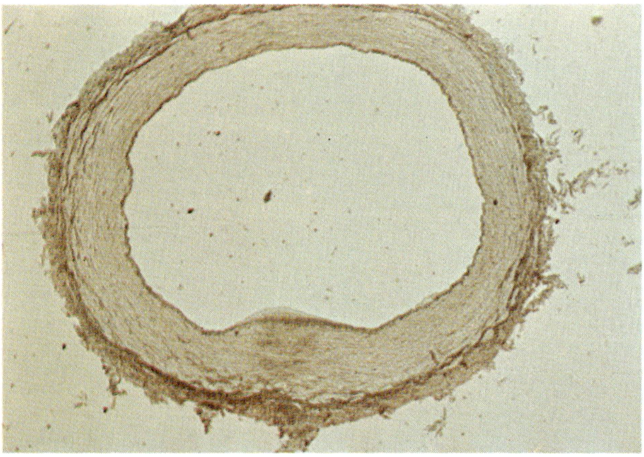

PLATE 29E

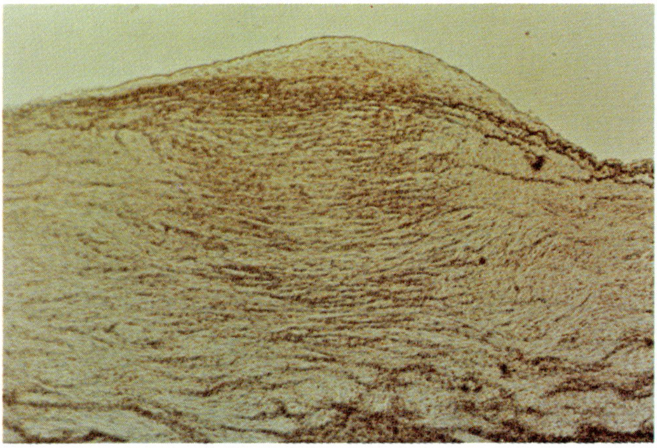

PLATE 29F

PLATE 22. Dog no. 5311. Curvature preparations—carotid artery to femoral artery autograft. Dates of surgery, 9/3/70–11/17/72 (26 months)—normal diet. Intimal proliferation at zones of curvature and suture attachment: (A) carotid artery to femoral artery autograft (left) producing curvatures—immediately postoperative; (B) carotid artery to femoral artery autograft (right) producing curvatures—immediately postoperative; (C) curvature preparation—26 months postoperative (left); (D) curvature preparation—26 months postoperative (right); (E) normal intima—note single layer of endothelium and internal elastic membrane; (F) intimal thickening—note normal internal elastic layer subjacent to intimal plaque; (G) intimal proliferation at site of suture fixation or attachment.

PLATE 23. Dog no. 2185. Dates of surgery, 9/15/61–9/25/63 (24 months)—normal diet: (A) curvature preparation—femoral artery to carotid artery autograft (24 months postoperative); (B) carotid artery with normal intima; (C) femoral artery—section from zone of curvature reveals intimal proliferation. (D) carotid artery with normal intima—medium power; (E) isometric femoral vein autograft to femoral artery (24 months postoperative); (F) femoral vein—shows intimal proliferation or plaque at zone of external attachment; (G) femoral vein—shows intimal proliferation at zone of external attachment; (H) femoral vein—showing intimal thickening by proliferation at zone of branching (ostial lesion). Note that blood flows as a branch rather than as a tributary.

PLATE 24. Dog no. 5278. Dates of surgery: 9/2/70–12/4/70 (3 months)—normal diet: (A) curvature produced by interposing a segment of carotid artery between ends of transected femoral artery (immediately postoperative); (B) same preparation 3 months later—note that curvatures have straightened due to longitudinal and circumferential contraction; (C) microscopic cross section reveals reduction of lumen by intimal and fibroblastic proliferation.

PLATE 25. Dog no. 2512. Carotid artery to femoral artery isometric graft. Dates of surgery: 10/5/62–12/20/63 (14 months)—normal diet: (A) surgical preparation immediately postoperative; (B) 14 months after surgery; (C) carotid artery showing concentric reduction of lumen by intimal and fibroblastic proliferation; (D) carotid artery showing further concentric reduction of lumen by intimal and fibroblastic proliferation; (E) carotid artery at a section distal to (D) showing obliteration of lumen by fibroblastic proliferation. Vessel is transformed into a fibrous cord; (F) microscopic section (high power) reveals remnants of internal elastic layer.

PLATE 26. Dog no. 1372. Curvature preparation—carotid artery to femoral artery autograft. Dates of surgery: 2/20/59–11/17/60 (21 months)—Specimens show intimal proliferation in carotid artery. Note absence of fat in intimal plaques: (A) femoral artery—normal—elastica stain; (B) carotid artery—concentric intimal proliferation, inspissated serum in lumen; (C) carotid artery—concentric intimal plaque—fat stain inspissated serum in lumen—note absence of fat in plaque; (D) Coronary artery (L.A.D.)—normal intima—trichrome stain; (E) coronary artery (L.A.D.)—normal intima—no plaque. Note fat in perivascular spaces and in muscle bundles; (F) kidney—fat stain—tubular cells show fatty infiltration.

PLATE 27. Dog no. 1261. Curvature preparation—carotid artery to femoral artery autograft. Dates of surgery: 12/12/58–5/27/60 (18 months)—normal diet: (A) femoral artery showing intimal proliferation.

Plaque is localized on convex wall of vessel seen here in cross section; (B) intimal plaque seen under higher magnification. Note intact internal elastic membrane; (C) intimal plaque—eccentrically localized—trichrome stain; (D) eccentric intimal proliferation—fat stain. Note absence of fat in plaque; (E) eccentric intimal plaque and intimal plaques or pads at orifice of a branch vessel; (F) intimal plaques or pads in ostial lesions. (See Figure 33.)

PLATE 28. Dog no. 1304. Curvature preparation—carotid artery to femoral artery autograft showing eccentric and concentric occlusive intimal proliferation. Plaques show both presence and absence of fat. Dates of surgery: 12/22/58–12/11/60 (24 months)—cholesterol fed: (A) carotid artery with concentric intimal proliferation—elastica stain; (B) carotid artery with concentric intimal proliferation—fat stain. Note absence of fat in plaque. Inspissated serum fills the lumen; (C) carotid artery—intimal fibroblastic proliferation almost totally occludes lumen—elastica stain; (D) carotid artery—eccentric plaque—with about 70% reduction of lumen—trichrome stain; (E) femoral artery—fat stain eccentric intimal proliferation with fat in the plaque and in media; (F) aorta—fat stain—dorsal wall shows fat in the intimal plaque and in the media (low power); (G) aorta—fat stain—shows fat in deeper zones of the intimal plaque; (H) coronary artery—trichrome stain—normal intima; (I) myocardium—fat stain—fatty infiltration of muscle tissue; (J) coronary artery—fat stain—no plaque, no fat in wall of vessel.

PLATE 29. Dog no. 1233A. Aortic narrowing (Venturi). Dates of surgery: 5/1/59–5/27/60 (12 months)—normal diet. Showing intimal proliferation containing fat at zone of suture fixation: (A) normal aorta; (B) aorta with intimal proliferation—plaque is localized to zone of suture fixation; (C) aortic intimal proliferation at zone of suture fixation; (D) aortic intimal proliferation at zone of external suture fixation; (E) aorta (fat stain) showing intimal plaque containing fat droplets (low power); (F) aorta—fat droplets in intimal plaque and subjacent media (medium power).

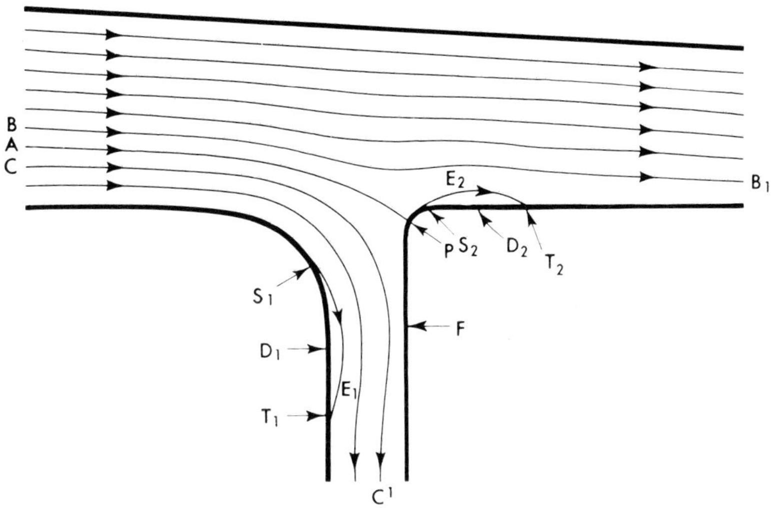

FIGURE 15. A qualitative sketch of streamlines expected where a small blood vessel (say 2 mm diameter) leaves a larger vessel (say 4 mm diameter) at right angles. At the stagnation point P, the shear stress is zero and the pressure will be a local maximum. The dividing streamline is AP; fluid above AP, such as BB′, remains in the parent vessel; fluid below AP, such as CC′, enters the daughter vessel. At the point S_1, a separation may occur and result in the formation of the eddy E_1. The pressure at D_1 will be at slightly lowered pressure due to the curvature of the streamline S_1T_1. Similarly, there may be a second eddy, E_2, with a separation point S_2 and a slightly lowered pressure point D_2 due to the curvature of the streamline S_2T_2. The point F may suffer a relatively high shear stress because of the higher velocity gradient there. From Texon (1972).

theoretically zero velocity (and zero shear stress) and is singularly free of atherosclerotic change. Because of the geometry in some cases, the streamlines of flow are forced to curve downstream of the stagnation point, giving rise to a local zone of increased velocity and probably lower pressure at point D_2 (Figure 15). A characteristic V-shaped lesion in the main stem distal to the branch is the localized biologic or reparative response to this flow pattern (Plate 5).

The pattern of blood flow into the orifice of a branch normal to the direction of main flow may produce, in effect, a tensile or suction force upon the wall (Plate 6).

BIFURCATION

Bifurcation lesion is the term applied to the intimal changes, including atherosclerotic plaques, that occur in the zone of bifurcation of a blood vessel. These lesions are here interpreted as the local biologic response of the blood vessel to hydraulic forces generated by the flowing blood. Although the patterns of flow at a bifurcation necessarily vary because of inherent variations in pulsatile flow as well as variations in geometry or anatomical design, idealized situations may be analyzed precisely and may serve as a basis for interpreting more complex patterns of flow.

The distribution of the pathological changes at a bifurcation reflects the predominant pattern of flow (Rodkiewicz and Roussel, 1973) as well as the gradual change in flow pattern due to the progressively developing anatomical lesion itself. The atherosclerotic plaque is, in effect, a composite result of all the pertinent hydraulic conditions. These chiefly include pulse rate, stroke volume, rhythm, pulsation, external attachment, amplitude, elasticity, ratio of the diameter of the trunk of the "Y" to the diameter of the branches, internal angle of branching, velocity of flow, and changes in velocity of flow.

The velocity distribution for streamline flow through a tube and an idealized bifurcation is shown diagrammatically in Figure 3. It is notable that the velocity of flow in a tube increases from the wall toward the center where it is a maximum. Division of the axial stream results in a relative increase in velocity and decrease in lateral pressure at the medial walls of the bifurcation branches, owing to the local curvatures required of the streamlines. In effect, the laws of fluid mechanics determine that the pattern of flow at a bifurcation is characterized by these two principal zones of diminished lateral pressure.

The precise sites of diminished lateral pressure (or suction effect) are determined in each instance by the velocity and curvatures of the streamlines of flow, that is, the pattern of flow as produced by the geometry or anatomical design, the flow pulse, and the viscosity of the blood.

Bifurcation of the Aorta and Common Iliac Arteries

The bifurcation of the aorta divides the central portion of blood flow. Under such hydraulic conditions a relative increase in velocity and decrease in lateral pressure are produced at the medial walls of the crotch zone compared with the lateral wall. These forces determine the medial walls of the crotch zone as sites of predilection for atherosclerotic changes (Plate 7). It is notable that the proximal margins of the atherosclerotic plaques in the common iliac arteries may be about 1 cm distal to the carina or the margin of the saddle of bifurcation. The carina and adjacent area, as stagnation zones, are singularly free of atherosclerotic change because of the local increase in pressure and theoretically zero velocity as well as zero shear stress at the point of impingement of blood flow. The increased pressure at the zone of impingement is less prone to produce atherosclerotic changes than the diminished lateral pressure at the immediately distal medial walls of the iliac arteries.

The angles of bifurcation (internal angle) of the common iliac arteries vary among different individuals (Plate 8). When the angle of bifurcation is relatively acute, the medial wall or crotch lesion develops (Plate 9). As the angle of bifurcation increases the lateral walls of the iliac arteries assume importance as inner walls of curvatures in continuity with the aorta. Under such conditions, a curvature lesion may develop on the lateral walls of the iliac arteries. The geometric pattern of the bifurcation will determine the hydraulic characteristics (Hung and Naff, 1969; Lynn et al., 1970) and sites of predilection for atherosclerotic change (Stehbens, 1975a) in each individual case.

Computational Simulation of Bifurcation Flow

This study is concerned with computing pressure, velocity, and wall shear stress in a bifurcation flow pattern to verify the existence and extent of areas of reduced pressure. While variations in the geometry could be introduced by different ratios of width of the branch vessels to parent vessel width and by different angles of branching, the geometry chosen here gives a typical flow pattern for the aortic bifurcation and representative computational results of two-dimensional, zero Reynolds number flow (Stokes flow). In the larger arteries there are local areas of turbulence (Stehbens, 1960), but for the purpose of calculating velocity and pressure distributions, Newtonian laminar flow is assumed. It is expected that this will not greatly affect the local pressures at low Reynolds numbers.

The finite element method (Davids and Cheng, 1972) is used by analyzing flow represented as two-dimensional viscous flow in an arterial bifurcation. As a first approximation, zero Reynolds number flow (Stokes flow) is assumed. Higher Reynolds number flows are treated as a second approximation including nonlinear terms. Numerical computations are made using the IBM 360 Computer.

Initially, the results of two-dimensional zero Reynolds number flow (Stokes flow) are obtained in a bifurcation (Figure 16)

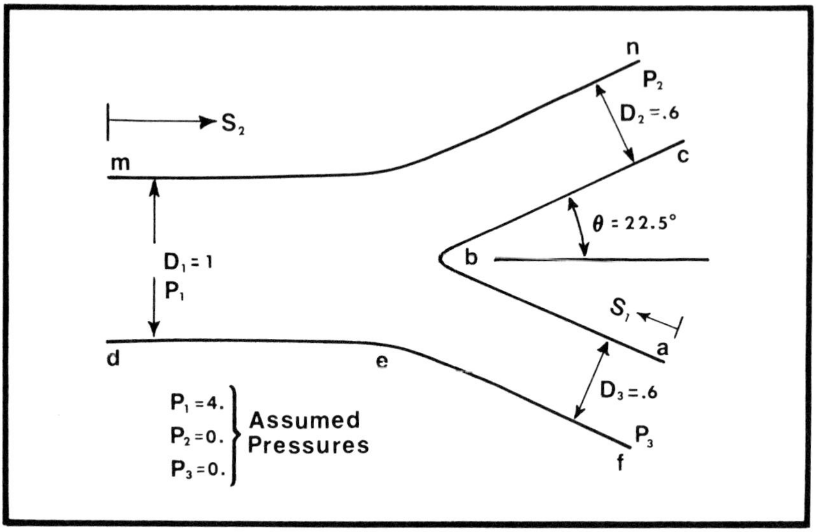

FIGURE 16. The geometry of an idealized bifurcation is considered. Dimensionless scales are used in presenting all computational results. The pressures and channel widths in dimensionless form are defined as follows: $P_1 = d_1 p_1 / \bar{V}\mu$, $P_2 = d_2 p_2 / \bar{V}\mu$, $P_3 = d_3 p_3 / \bar{V}\mu$; $D_1 = d_1/d_1$, $D_2 = d_2/d_1$, $D_3 = d_3/d_1$ where $\bar{V}$ = the mean approach velocity (cm/s), μ = viscosity of the fluid (dyn-s/cm^2 = poise), P = pressure (dyn/cm^2); d_1 = width of the entrance cross section md (cm); d_2 = width of the exit cross section nc (cm); d_3 = width of the exit cross section af (cm). From Texon (1976).

with a fixed upstream pressure and equal lower pressures in the downstream branches. Extension of the computer study includes calculations in a bifurcation with unequal pressures in the downstream branches. Computer programming for higher Reynolds number flows is in progress.

The typical finite element used in the coordinate plane (x,y) is shown in Figure 17A. Each edge of the element is located by two corner nodes and one side node to allow for curved sides. The curvilinear quadrilateral in (x,y) is mapped to the rectangle $\xi = \pm 1$, $\eta = \pm 1$ in the local coordinates ξ, η in Figure 17B by transformation (Ergatoudis et al., 1968; Skalak et al., 1970). The velocity components u and v in the x and y directions and the pressures are expressed by a similar approximation in terms of nodal values. Using unknown pressures at corner nodes and unknown velocities at all nodes leads to a system of about 300 simultaneous equations for a typical case to be solved simultaneously. Streamline distributions are also obtained by integration after computing the values of velocity components u and v.

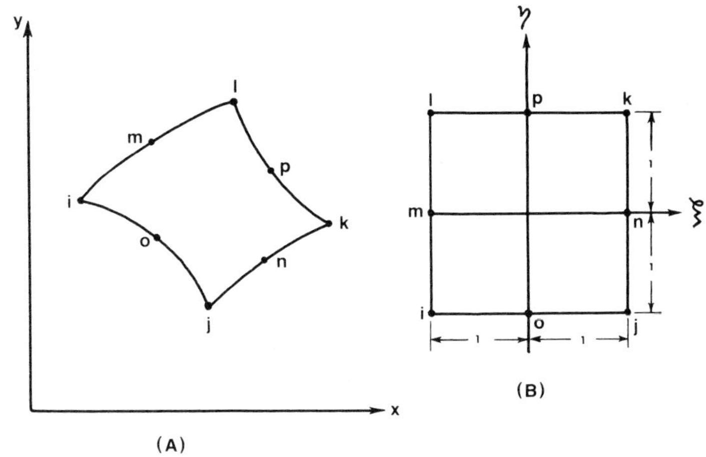

FIGURE 17. Finite element (A) in global coordinates x,y, and (B) in local coordinates ξ, η. From Skalak et al. (1970).

Results and Discussion

Two-dimensional zero Reynolds number bifurcation flows have been computed for the model shown in Figure 16. The corresponding streamline distributions are shown in Figure 18. There is a dividing streamline (shown dotted) that ends at the stagnation point on the wall. The fluid above and below the dividing streamline flows smoothly into one branch or the other without any separation of the flow from the wall. This is not unusual for low Reynolds number flows.

Figure 19 shows the pressure distributions (P_w) along the tube wall for the model bifurcation (Figure 16). The distances S_1 and S_2 are measured along the walls. Figure 19 shows that there are relatively low pressure areas at locations corresponding to the areas of predilection by atherosclerosis. These are the points marked A in Figure 19. Figures 20 and 21 show the wall shear stress (τ_w) along S_1 and S_2, respectively. The change of sign of τ_w indicates the physical fact that the shear stress changes direction at the stagnation point where its value is zero.

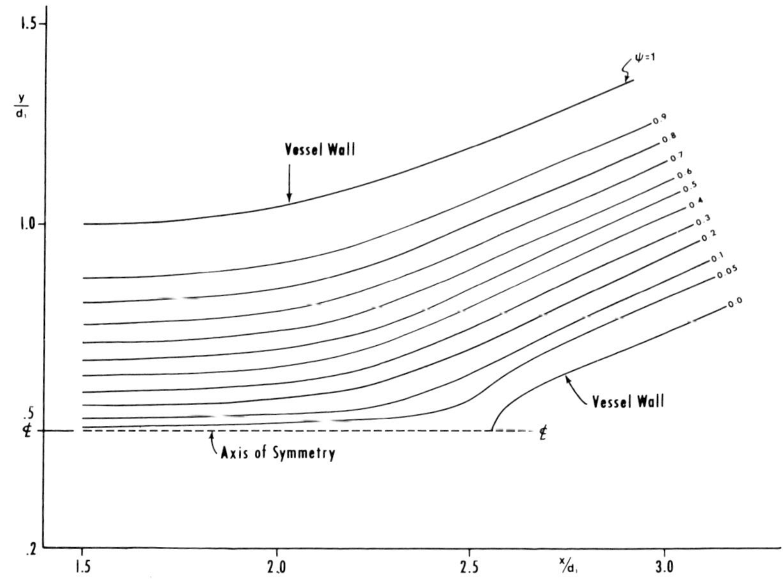

FIGURE 18. Streamlines for the geometric model shown in Figure 16. The values of the streamfunction shown on the diagram for each streamline are nondimensional and normalized by the total rate of flow as follows: In dimensional form, the streamfunction ψ is: $\psi = \int Vn\, dS$. In dimensionless form, the streamfunction ψ is defined as: $\psi = \psi / \overline{V} d_1$. The total rate of flow is $Q = \overline{V} d_1$. From Texon (1976).

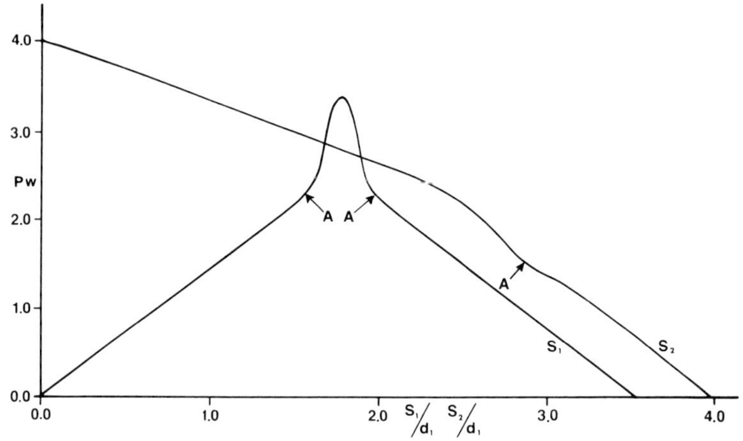

FIGURE 19. Wall pressure along the vessel wall plotted as a function of the distance S_1 and S_2 for the geometric model shown in Figure 16. The values of the pressure shown are nondimensionalized as follows: $\overline{P}_w = d_1 P_w / \overline{V} \mu$ where $\overline{V}$ = the mean approach velocity (cm/s), μ = viscosity of the fluid (dyn-s/cm^2 = poise), P_w = pressure on the vessel wall (dyn/cm^2), d_1 = width (cm) of the entrance cross section md in Figure 16, S_1 = the length (cm) along the vessel wall abc in Figure 16, S_2 = the length along the vessel wall def in Figure 16. From Texon (1976).

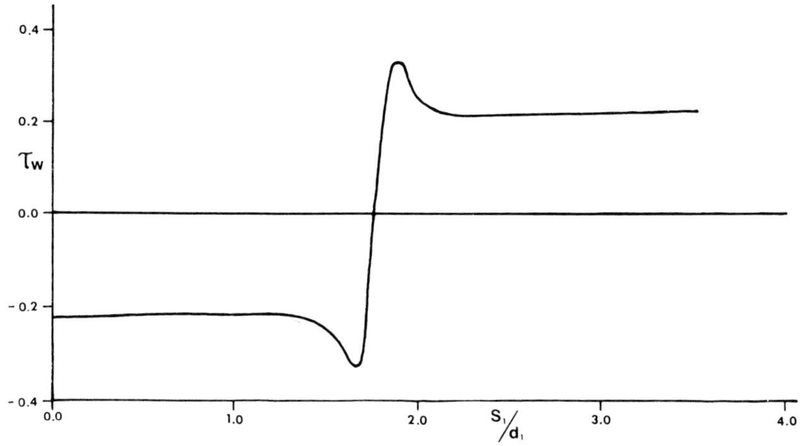

FIGURE 20. Wall shear stress along the vessel wall plotted as a function of the distance S_1 for the geometric model shown in Figure 16. The values of the wall shear stress shown in the diagrams are nondimensionalized as follows: In dimensional form the wall shear stress T_w is: $T_w = \mu\partial V/\partial n$. In dimensionless form the wall shear stress τ^w is defined as $\tau^w = Twd_1/\mu\bar{V}$ where d_1 = width (cm) of the entrance cross section md in Figure 16, μ = viscosity of the fluid (dyn-s/cm^2 = poise), $\bar{V}$ = mean approach velocity (cm/s), and V = velocity parallel to the wall, n = normal direction to the wall. From Texon (1976).

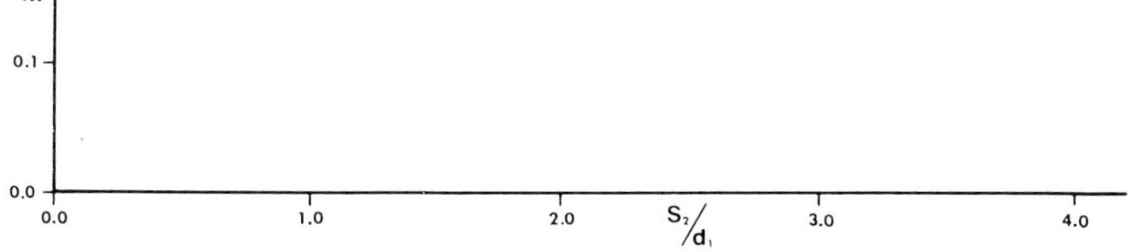

FIGURE 21. Wall shear stress along the vessel wall plotted as a function of the distance S_2 for the geometric model shown in Figure 16. The values of the wall shear stress shown in the diagrams are nondimensionalized as follows: In dimensional form the wall shear stress T_w is: $T_w = \mu\partial V/\partial n$. In dimensionless form the wall shear stress τ^w is defined as $\tau^w = Twd_1/\mu\bar{V}$ where d_1 = width (cm) of the entrance cross section md in Figure 16, μ = viscosity of the fluid (dyn-s/cm^2 = poise), $\bar{V}$ = mean approach velocity (cm/s), and V = velocity parallel to the wall, n = normal direction to the wall. From Texon (1976).

Thus, the foregoing indicates that relatively low pressure or suction areas can be discerned already at low Reynolds numbers. This effect may be expected to be enhanced and may also lead to regions of separation at higher Reynolds numbers. Such computations are currently being formulated. They require incorporation of the nonlinear terms of the Navier-Stokes equations and lead to considerably more involved computations.

Summary and Conclusion

Application of the laws of fluid mechanics to the natural conditions at the zone of aortic bifurcation reveals a rational and demonstrable basis for the localization, inception, and progressive development of atherosclerosis.

Computational simulation of bifurcation flow using the IBM 360 computer and the finite element method identifies low pressure areas even at two-dimensional zero Reynolds number flow. This effect is enhanced by higher Reynolds number flows. The low pressure areas show a definite correlation with the sites of predilection for the development of atherosclerosis. This study supports the conclusion that atherosclerosis may be considered the reactive biologic response of blood vessels to the effects of the mechanics of fluid flow, namely, the forces (diminished lateral pressure) generated by the flowing blood at the sites of predilection determined by local hydraulic characteristics in the circulatory system.

Trifurcation

The velocity distribution and flow pattern at a trifurcation are illustrated in Figure 22. The sites of predilection for atherosclerosis are demonstrated (Figure 23) to be the sites of relative diminution in pressure as determined in each instance by the relative velocities of flow at the wall of each branch, the angle of branching in relation to the curvature, the anatomical attachments and the ratio of trunk to branch diameter.

OTHER CONSIDERATIONS

In each of the above patterns of flow that relate to the anatomical design, an ideal geometry was described. Modifications of flow are produced by the natural asymmetry or imperfections in the anatomic geometry of the blood vessels. Further modifications are produced progressively as the atherosclerotic process influences the velocity and volumetric flow by encroachment on the lumen.

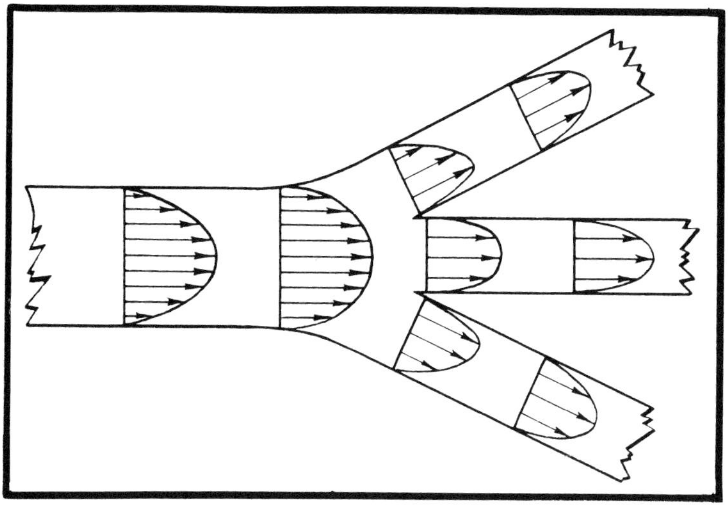

FIGURE 22. Velocity distribution for laminar flow along a tube and at a trifurcation. From Texon (1963).

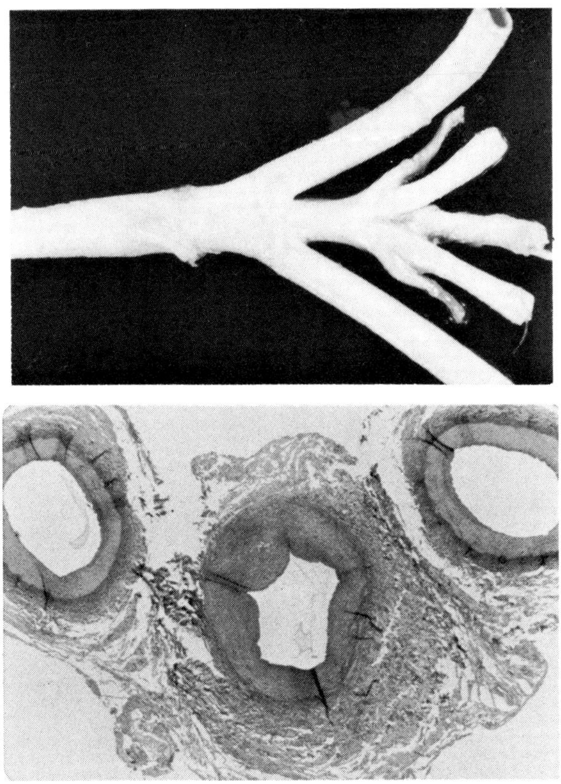

FIGURE 23. (Top) Dog, trifurcation of the aorta—gross specimen. (Bottom) Dog, intimal thickening at sites of predilection in a trifurcation of aorta—microscopic specimen.

It should be emphasized that several hydraulic conditions may be found concurrently. Thus, a tapering vessel may at the same time branch or have an attachment, etc. The composite effect of all the local hydraulic specifications (i.e., curvature, taper, branch, bifurcation, and attachment) will influence the velocity of flow and lateral pressure at a given site with respect to its predilection for atherosclerotic change.

7 HUMAN ATHEROSCLEROSIS

VASCULAR EMBRYOLOGY AND SUBSEQUENT DEVELOPMENT (THE REPARATIVE RESPONSE)

The vascular system develops embryologically by means of endothelial sprouts from an early capillary network formed by the growth and coalescence of blood islands in the mesoderm. The vascular outgrowths are guided in their course by epithelial obstructions that determine the position of the capillary plexuses. Favorable channels enlarge and become main arteries and veins sending forth new branches. The hydraulic characteristics change both generally and locally while the anatomic design elaborates in response to the growth needs of the organism as a whole and the needs of individual organs. Hydraulic conditions conducive to atherosclerosis appear *in utero* as soon as blood begins to flow in definitive channels. The anatomic design of the vascular system and the natural laws of fluid mechanics provide hydraulic specifications that are prerequisite and conducive to atherosclerosis. The earliest lesions, intimal thickening, are found at certain sites of predilection, namely, regions of relative decrease in lateral pressure such as are produced by curvature, tapering, bifurcation, branching, or external attachments. The continuous operation of local hydraulic forces throughout life makes further pathological changes inherently possible. In fact, atherosclerosis, as a progressive occlusive arterial disease, or its pathological complications, is a major cause of human disability and death.

ILLUSTRATIVE EXAMPLES

The human circulatory system is necessarily characterized by specific hydraulic-biologic conditions. The precise correlation of atherosclerotic lesions with their localization at sites of predilection, namely, regions of diminished lateral pressure, in accordance with the laws of fluid mechanics is demonstrated by the examples that follow.

The Coronary Circulation

The coronary circulation is unique with respect to its hydraulic characteristics. The flow of blood is intermittent as a result of systolic contraction of the heart. The blood stream is subject to abrupt, rapid, and wide fluctuations in velocity, increased velocity and volumetric flow occurring during diastole, and reduced velocity and volumetric flow occurring during systole. Retrograde or reversal of flow under certain conditions also occurs. The coronary arteries are unique in the body with respect to such wide phasic variations in blood flow. It is notable that the caliber of the extramural coronary arteries tapers rapidly. The anatomic curvatures inherent in the coronary

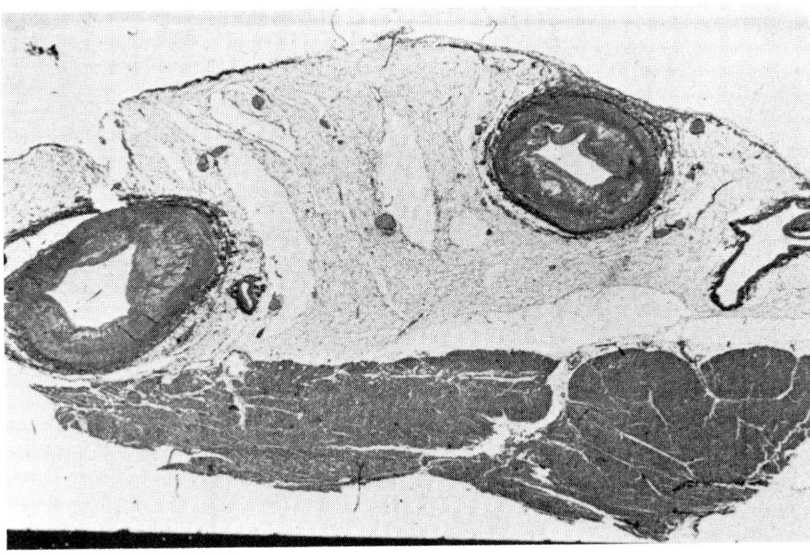

FIGURE 24. Human coronary atherosclerosis—showing concentric occlusive disease in a relatively free and straight portion of left anterior descending branch—a "converging boundary" or "taper" lesion. From Texon (1963).

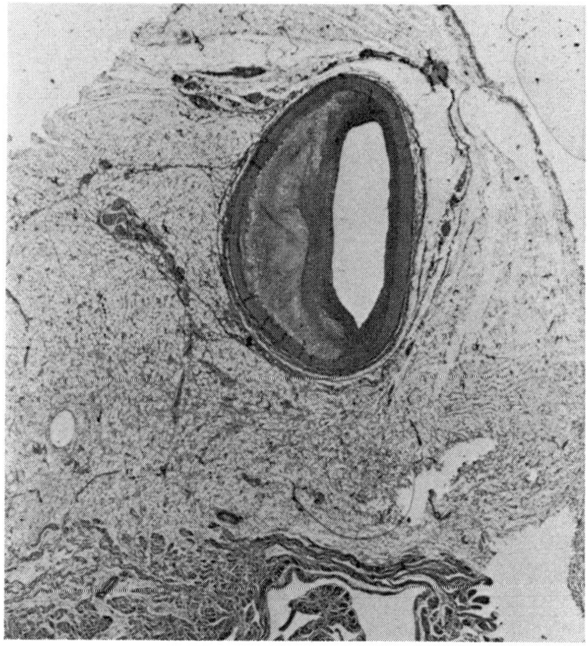

FIGURE 25. Human coronary atherosclerosis–showing eccentric occlusive disease in a "curvature" lesion–right coronary artery at acute margin of heart. From Texon (1957). Copyright 1957, American Medical Association.

circulation are also notable. The composite effect of these hydraulic factors (namely, the rapid changes in velocity of flow, the nozzle effect of tapering, and the inherent anatomical curves) seem to be significant factors in the predisposition of the coronary arteries toward atherosclerotic changes. Pathological examination of coronary arteries reveals uniformly that the atherosclerotic process develops at sites of predilection that are determined by the local hydraulic conditions. A free and straight vessel presents correspondingly more concentric atherosclerotic change (Figure 24). The forces generated by blood flow in a zone of curvature determine a greater degree of involvement of the inner (convex) wall compared with the outer wall (Figure 25). The free epicardial aspect of a coronary artery may be less affected by atherosclerotic change than the tethered or attached surface. The reduced lumen at the site of atherosclerosis due to curvature or attachment will be, of necessity, eccentrically placed. A frequent finding is a segmental linear atherosclerotic plaque involving the left coronary artery beginning approximately 1 cm from its origin at a zone where it curves and continues to form the left anterior descending branch (Plate 10). This is a curvature lesion aptly described as a "waterfall" lesion.

The Aorta

The predilection of the aortic arch for atherosclerotic changes and dissecting hematomas is determined by the high velocity of blood flow and reduced static pressure or suction effect that characterize the hydraulic specifications in this region. A common finding is a large atherosclerotic plaque (Plate 11) on the inner curvature of the aortic arch, a "sentinel patch." The sudden release of intraabdominal pressure in the Valsalva maneuver causes a sudden increase in aortic blood velocity. The accompanying suction effect due to the sudden diminution in lateral pressure may tear the aortic wall by overcoming the bond between the layers to produce a dissecting hematoma (Figure 26). One of the earliest plaques to appear is located at the obliterated exit of the ductus arteriosus, an "attachment" lesion. The thoracic aorta typically and invariably presents atherosclerotic changes predominantly on the dorsal surface (Plates 11 and 12). Tapering of the aorta and effects of gravity result in a relative increase in blood velocity in the abdominal portion of the aorta with consequently more severe atherosclerosis in this area. In advanced instances of atherosclerosis of the aorta, the involvement may be diffuse, affecting both dorsal and ventral walls.

Bifurcation of the Aorta and Common Iliac Arteries

The bifurcation of the aorta divides the more central streamlines. Under such hydraulic conditions a relative increase in velocity and decrease in lateral pressure are produced at the medial walls of the crotch zone compared with the lateral walls. These forces determine the medial walls of the crotch zone as sites of predilection for atherosclerotic changes (Figure 27). It is notable that the proximal margins of the atherosclerotic plaques in the common iliac arteries may be about 1 cm distal to the carina or the margin of bifurcation (Plate 13). This area, as a stagnation point, is free of atherosclerosis because of the local increase in pressure where impingement of the blood stream occurs. The high impingement pressure is less prone to produce atherosclerotic changes than the diminished lateral pressure at the immediately distal medial walls of the crotch zone.

It may be noted that the angles of bifurcation of the

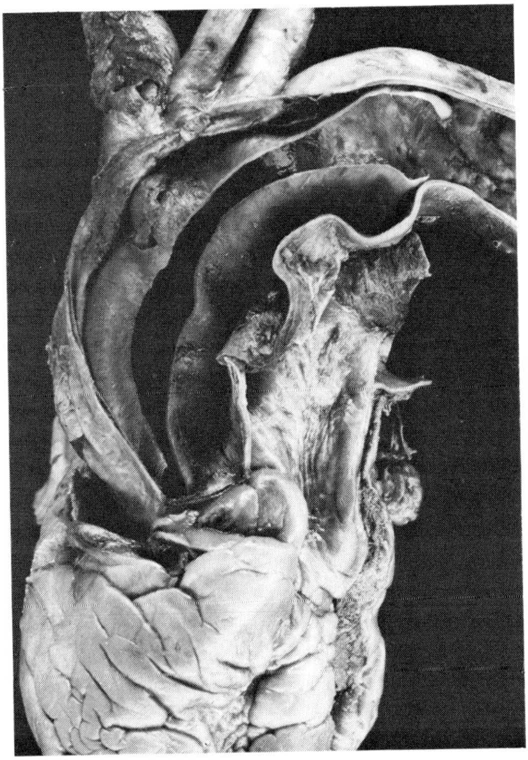

FIGURE 26. Dissecting hematoma involving entire aortic arch (see text). From Burchell (1955), by permission of the American Heart Association, Inc.

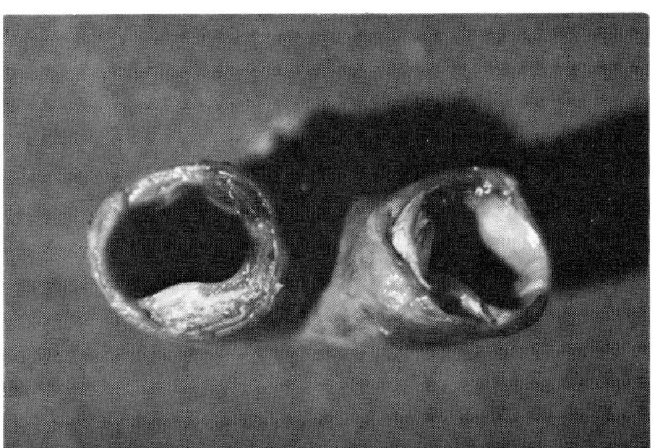

FIGURE 27. Black woman, age 62, bifurcation of the aorta. Note atherosclerotic thickening of medial walls of the common iliac arteries. From Texon (1976a).

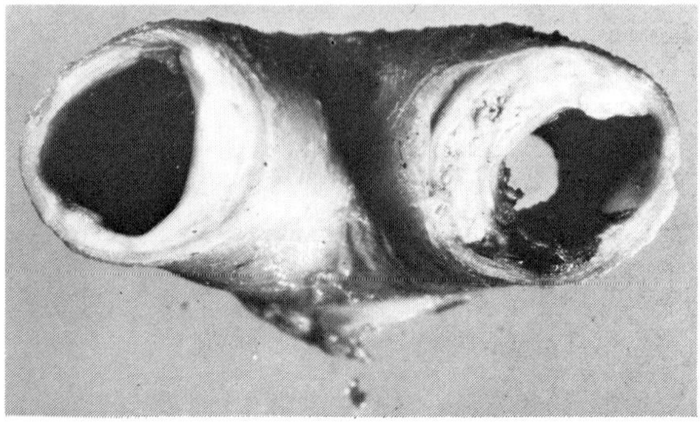

FIGURE 28. Bifurcation of the aorta showing atherosclerotic thickening of medial walls of the iliac arteries (see Plate 8). From Texon (1957). Copyright 1957, American Medical Association.

common iliac arteries vary among different individuals (Figure 28). When the angle of bifurcation is relatively acute (Figure 29) the medial wall or crotch lesion develops. As the angle of bifurcation increases the lateral walls of the iliac arteries assume their anatomic importance as convex walls of curvatures in continuity with the aorta. Under such conditions, curvature

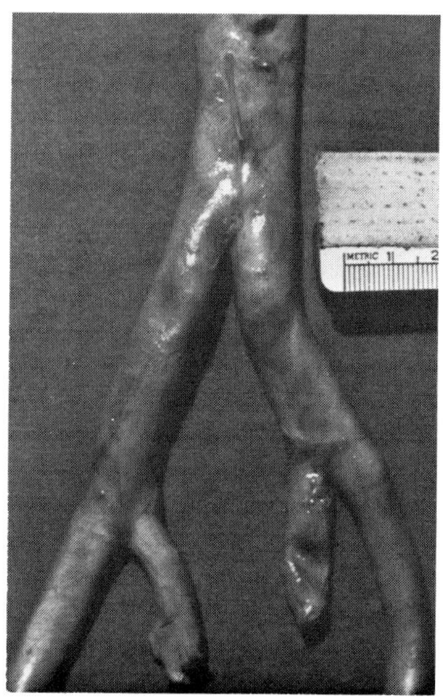

FIGURE 29. Terminal aorta, bifurcation, common iliac arteries with internal and external iliac branches—gross specimen (see Figure 27).

lesions may appear on the lateral walls of the iliac arteries. The geometry or anatomic design of the aortic bifurcation will determine the hydraulic characteristics and sites of predilection for atherosclerosis in each individual.

Splenic Arteries

The splenic artery is remarkable for its tortuosity and relatively large caliber. The large caliber serves to decrease the velocity of the blood flow. Atherosclerosis is therefore less frequent. Nevertheless, atherosclerosis is found as a result of the local hydraulic characteristics in accordance with the laws of fluid mechanics. An atherosclerotic plaque is noted on the inner walls of the curvatures in the specimen illustrated (Plate 14).

Ostial or Branch Lesions

Ostial lesion is the term applied to the intimal changes, including atherosclerotic plaques, that occur at the zone of origin of a branch vessel. These lesions are here interpreted as the local biologic response of the blood vessel to hydraulic forces generated by the flowing blood. Although the patterns of flow at a branch necessarily vary because of variations in pulsatile flow as well as variations in geometry or anatomical design, idealized situations may be analyzed precisely and may serve as a basis for interpreting more complex patterns of flow. The distribution of the pathological changes reflects the predominant pattern of flow as well as the change in pattern of flow due to the progressively developing anatomical lesion itself. The atherosclerotic plaque is, in effect, the composite result of all the pertinent hydraulic conditions. These may include pulse rate, stroke volume, rhythm, amplitude, elasticity, ratio of the diameter of the main stem to branch diameter, shape of the ostial orifice, angle of branching, and velocity of flow.

The laws of fluid mechanics determine that the pattern of flow at the site of a branch is usually characterized by several zones of diminished lateral pressure. These may be identified at points D_1 and D_2 (Figure 15). The relatively high shear stress at point F reflects the increased velocity gradient adjacent to the wall surface or at the interface.

It is notable that in any branching anatomical pattern a stagnation point must develop at the distal margin of the ostial orifice. The stagnation point is a point of high pressure and theoretically zero velocity (and zero shear stress) and is singularly free of atherosclerotic change. Because of the geometry in some cases, the streamlines of flow are forced to curve downstream of the stagnation point, giving rise to a local zone of increased velocity and probably lower pressure at point D_2 (Figure 15). A characteristic V-shaped lesion in the main stem distal to the branch is the localized biologic or reparative response to this flow pattern (Plate 15 and Figure 30).

The pattern of blood flow into the orifice of a branch normal to the direction of main flow may produce, in effect, a tensile or suction force upon the wall (Plate 16).

Comment

Zones of branching give rise to ostial lesions. They are examples of sites of predilection for atherosclerosis—localized areas of diminished pressure where the endothelium is exposed to the lifting or pulling effect and tensile stress exerted by the flowing blood. This is the initial stimulus. The initial response is a biologic change, a reparative or reactive thickening due to the proliferation of intimal cells. There is no evidence of hematological (blood) reaction, lipid change, or vascularization in the early stage of intimal thickening. The internal elastic layer appears to remain intact and unchanged in the early lesions.

With continuing blood flow, the thickening intima encroaches upon the lumen. The plaque progresses in size, shape, and degree, with further pathological change depending upon the pattern of blood flow and the zones of varying diminution in lateral pressure. The pathological process may also be the biologic response at the wall to the effect of increased shear stress at the interface. The varying successive hydraulic stresses may be reflected in the orientation of cells in successive layers of fibroblastic proliferation. While fibroblastic proliferation appears to be the dominant pathological change at all stages, cellular elements and lipids are added to the intimal and fibroblastic proliferation as part of the pathological response *in situ.*

Summary

The influences of fluid mechanics have been reviewed with special reference to patterns of flow in the region of the orifice of a branching blood vessel. The traumatic (pathological) effects are associated with zones of low pressure, zones of increased shear stress, and zones of increased velocity gradient. Intimal proliferation associated with an ostial orifice is demonstrated to be the biologic response to the tensile stress created by the flowing blood at low pressure zones determined by the ana-

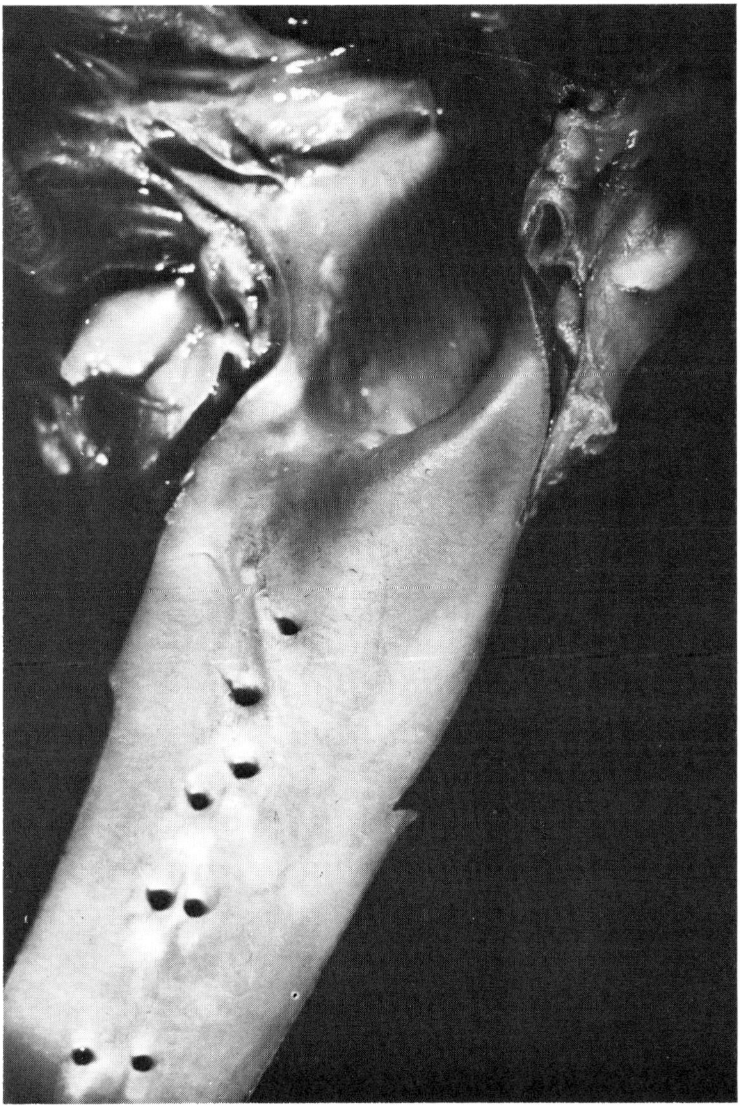

FIGURE 30. Dog (normal diet), ostial lesions in aorta, distal to orifices of intercostal arteries. From Texon (1972).

tomical pattern. The ostial lesion is here interpreted to be the biologic response of the blood vessels to the mechanical stimulus (diminished lateral pressure) inherent in the effect of the laws of hemodynamics as they apply to local hydraulic specifications in the zone of origin of a branch vessel.

Arteriovenous Fistulas

The experimental production of arteriovenous fistulas (Baumann et al., 1976) and pathological findings in the clinical use of arteriovenous fistulas (Stehbens, 1968; Stehbens and Karmody, 1975) confirm the development of arterial atherosclerosis and venous atherosclerosis as a response to the localized increase in blood velocity, although altered endothelial permeability and vibrational effects have been implicated.

Pulmonary Artery

The pulmonary ring and pulmonary artery have a greater circumference than the aortic ring and ascending aorta. Normally, the same volume of blood per unit time must pass these sections; thus, the velocity of flow is lower in the pulmonary artery compared with the velocity of flow in the ascending aorta. Therefore, atherosclerosis due to the suction effect of the blood stream is uncommon or minimized in the pulmonary artery.

Veins

Veins present gradually diverging lines of flow and have a larger caliber than corresponding arteries. The velocity of blood flow is relatively low and comparatively steady in veins (Figure 31). The suction effect upon the walls of veins is therefore minimal, and occlusive sclerotic changes are comparatively rare.

Ductus Arteriosus

The ductus arteriosus and umbilical vessels provide examples of transformations of blood vessels into fibrotic cords as a response to changes in local hydraulic conditions.

In a vessel of fixed diameter the volumetric blood flow is directly proportional to the velocity of blood flow ($Q = AV$). A velocity of flow above the ideal physiological limit is conducive to the production of segmental zones of diminished lateral pressure with resultant intimal proliferation and further atherosclerotic changes at the sites of predilection. Conversely, a velocity of blood flow and lateral pressure below a critical level may fail to maintain adequate mechanical patency of the lumen because of elasticity or external pressure, and intimal proliferation may then encroach upon the lumen (Plates 17, 18, 19). In some instances external pressure or twisting of a blood vessel partially occludes the lumen and diminishes the blood flow to such a degree that intimal proliferation may further encroach

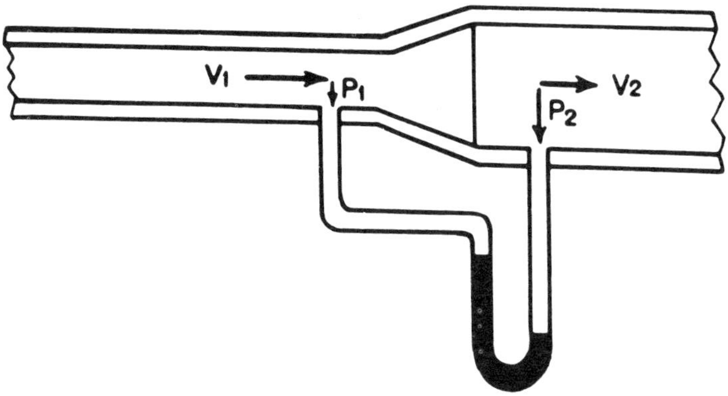

FIGURE 31. Diagram of diverging walls, pressure, and velocity changes as found in veins (see text.) From Texon (1971).

upon the lumen and even transform the vessel into a fibrotic cord.

Consider a blood vessel with a normal pressure and velocity of blood flow. The diameter will vary between normal limits depending on the systolic and diastolic pressure in the vessel. If, at a given site, the blood flow is permanently altered by disease, external pressure, or by surgical intervention so that the systolic and diastolic pressures are reduced, both the diameter and length of the vessel distally will be correspondingly reduced by the contraction of the elastic tissue in the wall. If the blood flow is still further reduced so that, despite a maximum reduction in diameter and length resulting from contraction of elastic tissue fibers, patency of the lumen cannot be maintained by the blood pressure, the lumen collapses or becomes gradually obliterated by endothelial and fibroblastic proliferation. This process should not be considered a form of atherosclerosis but rather a reparative biologic or cellular response that serves to occlude an unused lumen and to transform the vessel into a fibrous cord. This appears to be a mechanism for the occlusion of bypass grafts, namely, intimal and fibroblastic proliferation secondary to diminished blood flow. It is of particular interest and importance to vascular surgeons.

It is apparent that a normal physiological range of blood volume requires a normal range of pressure and velocity of blood flow to minimize intimal proliferation due to either excessively high blood velocity or excessively low blood velocity.

8 EXPERIMENTAL ATHEROSCLEROSIS IN DOGS

AIM OF EXPERIMENTS

An approach to scientific proof that the effect of the laws of fluid mechanics is the primary causative factor in the etiology and pathogenesis of atherosclerosis may be achieved by altering hydraulic characteristics under controlled conditions in order to observe changes in the arterial wall (Texon et al., 1960; Texon et al., 1962; Imparato et al., 1961).

METHOD

Anatomical and hydraulic conditions of the experiment are designed to simulate those operating in human blood vessels with respect to curvilinear flow, flow in a tapering blood vessel, flow at sites of branching, and flow at sites of fixation or external attachment.

1. S-shaped curvatures are produced surgically by interposing an excised section of carotid artery as an autograft between the ends of the transected femoral artery. The femoral artery becomes elongated by the autograft and assumes variable S-shaped configurations.
2. Similarly, S-shaped curvatures are produced surgically by interposing an excised section of femoral artery as an autograft between the ends of the transected carotid artery. The carotid artery becomes elongated by the autograft and assumes variable S-shaped configurations.

3. In some cases the curvatures after variable intervals of time are restored to relatively straight configurations by virtue of their longitudinal contracture, circumferential contracture, and external attachment, with corresponding changes in blood flow patterns and arterial wall changes.
4. Arterial wall changes are observed and documented at sites of branching, tapering, bifurcation, trifurcation, external attachment, and sites of surgical sutures.
5. The effect on the wall of isometric arterial grafts is noted.
6. The effect of blood flow patterns is noted on the intima of veins when a section of vein is interposed as an autograft between the transected ends of an artery.
7. Control sections of all vessels are taken at the time of surgery and compared with sections examined after the dogs are fed a normal kennel ration for 6 to 36 months.
8. Vessels of dogs fed a high cholesterol diet are also examined.

Experimental methods and findings discussed in this section are illustrated in the experimental protocols (Experimental Protocol Plates 21–29, Figure 32).

FINDINGS

Gross Observations

The surgically altered femoral and carotid arteries including the carotid and femoral autografts are found to be patent, pulsating, and to have assumed varying forms of S-shaped curvatures with attachments to adjacent tissue. The intact sections are photographed *in situ,* excised, and examined histologically.

Some S-shaped surgical preparations are found to have become relatively straight due to longitudinal contracture, circumferential contracture, and external fixation. The vessels appear to be without pulse and transformed to fibrotic cords.

Microscopic Observations

A single layer of endothelium overlying an intact internal elastic layer is the basic finding in the normal artery and vein. All control sections of carotid and femoral arteries are found to be normal.

The endothelial lining consisting of a single layer of cells represents the initial thickness of the intima. Both the intima

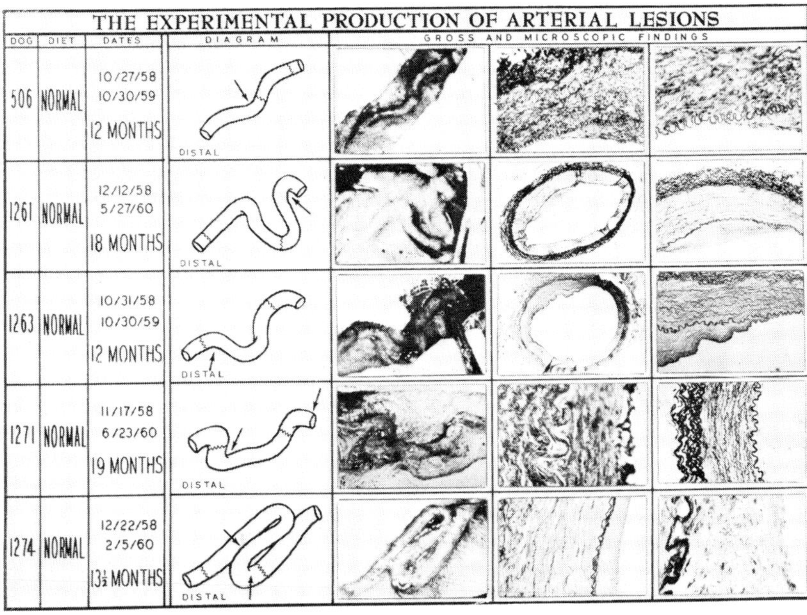

FIGURE 32. Hemodynamically induced arterial lesions in dogs. Arrows indicate sites of microscopic sections illustrated. Note: Arterial wall changes are observed in five dogs maintained on a normal kennel ration for 12–19 months after the surgical production of S-shaped curvatures. The arterial wall lesions consist of intimal plaques localized at the internal (convex) wall of the curvatures and at zones of external attachment. The histological changes consist of fibroblastic proliferation of the intima with intact endothelial and internal elastic layers. From Texon et al. (1962). Copyright 1962, American Medical Association.

and internal elastic layer are intact and unchanged in the normal arterial wall. The earliest change is a thickening of the intima by proliferation of the endothelium and subjacent cells—to form a localized intimal plaque. There is an absence of inflammatory cellular infiltration, vascularization, and lipid formation in the early lesions. The intimal proliferation and fibroblastic proliferation become the earliest atherosclerotic plaque with localization at specific sites of predilection characterized by lower wall pressure (tensile stress) in accordance with the effect of the laws of fluid mechanics and a local pattern of blood flow.

The earliest lipid change is noted in the form of minute droplets within fibroblasts in the basement zone of the intima. More advanced lesions reveal lipid droplets that coalesce and extend toward the luminal surface. Fibroblastic proliferation is the predominant change.

In a curvature lesion, the thickened intima assumes a crescentic shape with the greatest thickness corresponding to the convex wall of the curvature. This is an eccentric atherosclerotic plaque. In a taper lesion the intima thickens more uniformly to form a concentric atherosclerotic plaque. In some lesions capillary revascularization is noted. Instances of intramural intimal hemorrhage have also been seen.

At zones of suturing a cellular response is noted in addition to the intimal and fibroblastic proliferation. The fibroblastic response not only restores the structural integrity of the interrupted media and adventia but also produces intimal thickening that gradually encroaches on the lumen of the vessel. In some cases intimal proliferation produces tongue-like projections into the lumen. In other cases intimal proliferation extends across the lumen producing subdivision of the channel and a multiluminal appearance.

Transformation of a blood vessel into a fibrotic cord occurs when blood flow is progressively diminished by local hydraulic conditions.

DISCUSSION

Application of the laws of fluid mechanics to the altered vascular configurations produced surgically in dogs reveals vascular changes comparable in every way to atherosclerosis as it occurs in humans. Segmental intimal proliferation with progressively occlusive pathological changes occurs consistently at sites of predilection in the circulatory system. These include curvatures, tapering, bifurcation, trifurcation, external attachment, and branching. As previously pointed out, the common feature of blood flow in these configurations is the diminished lateral pressure, or tensile force, generated at some phase of the pulsatile flow. This tensile force or suction effect tends to move the wall inward toward the axial stream and stimulates the single layer of endothelium to proliferate and thicken. The thickened intima and its progressive pathological changes are the atherosclerotic plaques.

It is noteworthy that dogs fed a normal diet may present atherosclerotic plaques with and without fat in the lesions. Similarly, dogs fed a cholesterol diet may present atherosclerotic plaques with and without fat in the lesions. It must be concluded that fats are not a causative factor in atherosclerosis.

Fat in the atherosclerotic plaque is part of an *in situ* pathological or reparative change.

The constancy of the findings in all the experimental preparations and the application of the pertinent laws of fluid mechanics support the conclusion that the effect of the laws of fluid mechanics, vascular dynamics, is the primary causative factor in the localization, inception, and progressive development of atherosclerosis.

9 HYDRAULIC MODEL FINDINGS

Glass models that simulate hydraulic conditions in the circulatory system provide confirmation of the existence, location, and magnitude of low pressure areas at sites of curvature, tapering, branching, and bifurcation. Despite the effects that elasticity and pulsatile flow impose on wall pressure, wall shear stress, and velocity of flow, the basic findings in rigid glass models with steady flow and in similar models with pulsatile flow show a precise correlation between low pressure zones and the sites of predilection for the development of atherosclerosis.

10 DISCUSSION AND CONCLUSIONS

BLOOD FLOW–A LIFE REQUIREMENT

Atherosclerosis, beginning with intimal proliferation, is an ongoing process that appears *in utero* as soon as blood begins to flow in definite channels. The continuous operation of local hydraulic forces throughout life makes further pathological changes inherently possible. Atherosclerosis is a price we pay for blood flow as a requirement of life. Atherosclerotic lesions are consistently found at sites of predilection at all ages. The severity of the process does not bear a linear relation to age but rather to time in relation to local hydraulic specifications (Plate 20, Figure 33). The fact is that atherosclerosis as a progressive arterial disease and its pathological complications are a major cause of human illness, disability, and death.

STIMULUS VS. RESPONSE

While the development of atherosclerosis must depend upon the operation of its primary etiologic factor (local diminution in lateral pressure produced at sites of predilection by the effects of flowing blood) the rate of development and severity of the disease may be modified by biologic factors. It is here that genetic tissue differences in reactive or reparative response to injury at the cellular level may determine the nature and degree of atherosclerotic change in each individual.

The Reparative Response

Arterial endothelium (Balint, 1974) is a monocellular layer whose individual cells have a limited life span. The replacement

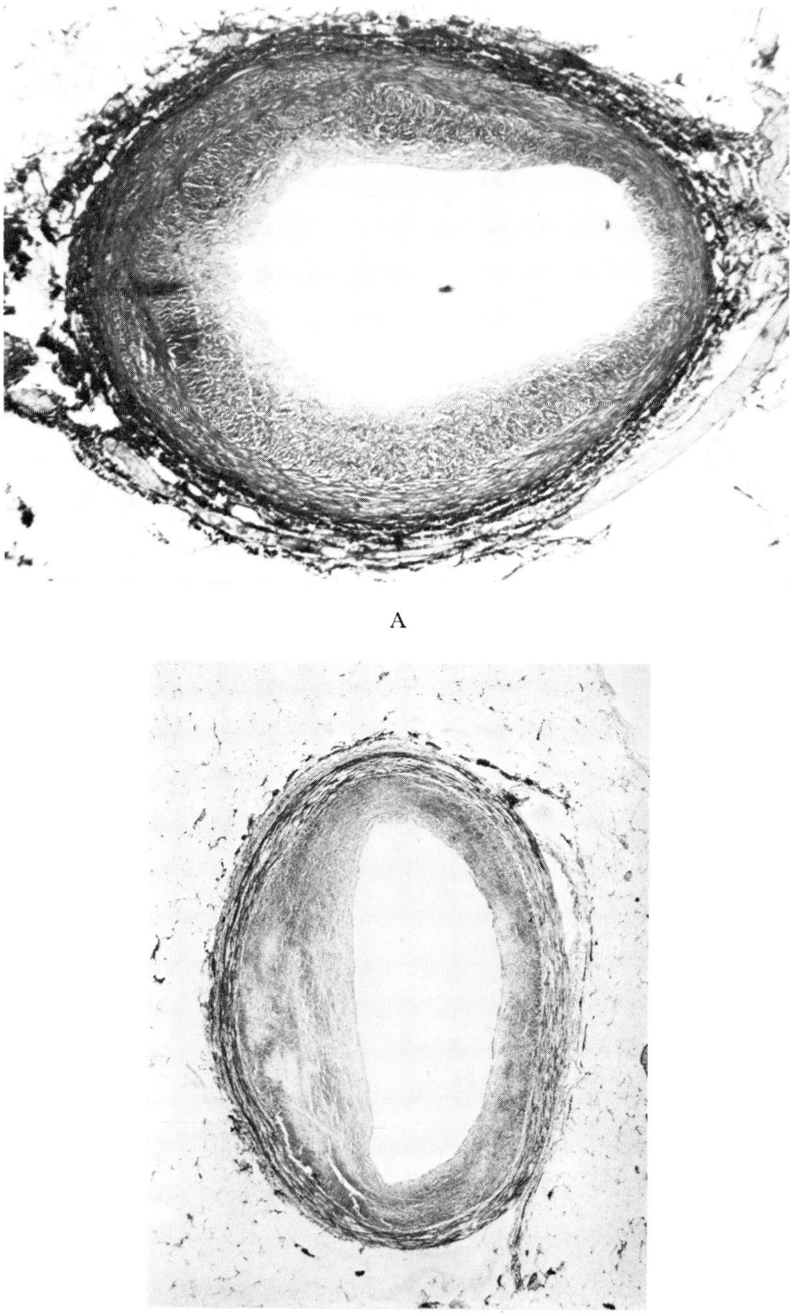

B

FIGURE 33. (A) Black male, age 5 months, coronary artery (L.A.D.). Note eccentric intimal thickening in a "curvature" lesion. From Texon (1976). (B) White male, age 56, coronary artery (L.A.D.). From Texon (1974).

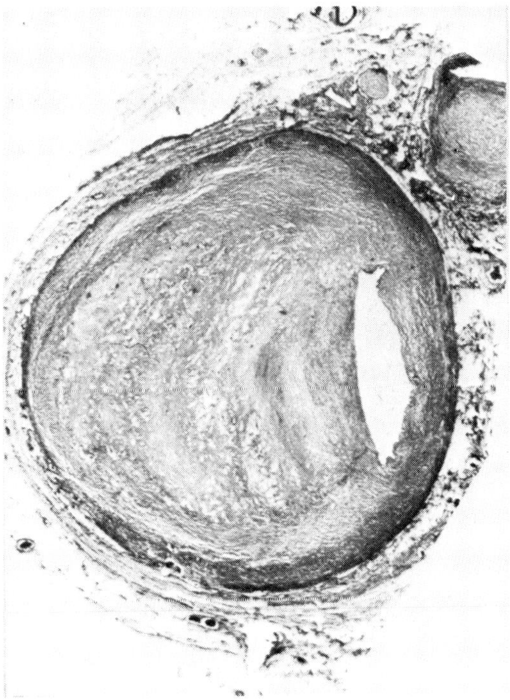

C

FIGURE 33. (*Continued*) (C) White woman, age 29, coronary artery (L.A.D.). Note that reduction in lumen by atherosclerosis does not bear a linear relation to chronological age. (See text.) From Texon (1974).

of loosened, shrunken, and desquamated endothelial cells occurs by extension and division of surrounding endothelial cells. The turnover may be constant for a given area but varies from one arterial segment to another and is particularly increased in areas exposed to greater hemodynamic stresses (Glagov, 1972), such as curvatures, branchings, and bifurcations. Medial smooth muscle cells may constitute the cellular elements of the intimal proliferation in pathological processes and substitute for deteriorated endothelial cells. They may play a role in the production of extracellular substances such as collagen, elastica, and basement membrane. Vascular smooth muscle cells thus resemble primordial mesenchymal cells (Wissler, 1967) capable of responding to altered circumstances by change in shape and function.

Regeneration of endothelium follows upon many forms of injury (Veress et al., 1969), the mode and rate depending on the extent of denudation (Fishman et al., 1975), the species, and the cumulative physical effect of the tensile stress exerted on the vessel wall by velocity of the flowing blood as determined by the local vascular configuration (Baumann et al., 1976; Fry, 1968; Imparato et al., 1974). Kern et al. (1972) concluded that intimal fibrosis represents a reparative phenomenon in response to hemodynamic stress. The proliferation of arterial endothelium may be seen to grow over a prosthesis or cover a thrombus at a site of underlying destruction of endothelium.

It is recognized that normal endothelium maintains a selective bidirectional permeability (Jellinek, 1974; Smith et al., 1976) to nutrients and metabolites (Chernick et al., 1949) for the arterial wall (Caro et al., 1971; Caro, 1973) while at the same time maintaining its own structural integrity (Fry, 1973) despite the constant motion inherent in pulsatile flow.

The proliferation of endothelium (Altschul, 1954; Haust, 1976; Haust et al., 1959) that is initially a single layer of cells adjacent to the internal elastic layer gives rise to a multilayered intima that lies between the endothelium and the internal elastic layer. The thickened intima, with progressive *in situ* changes due to further differentiation of endothelial cells, proliferation of fibroblasts and smooth muscle cells (Benditt and Benditt, 1973; Geer and Haust, 1972; Ross, 1973; Thomas et al., 1963), and precipitation of lipid elements, becomes the well-defined atherosclerotic plaque (Mitchell and Schwartz, 1965; Wissler, 1974).

An early stage in fibroatheromatous plaque formation may be postulated: the local increase in tensile stress (diminished lateral pressure), acting as the primary stimulus, causes an altered permeability (French, 1966) of the endothelium and intima with a proliferation of smooth muscle cells, fibroblasts, and collagen (Friedman et al., 1975); More, 1973). A gelatinous or insudation lesion results from the excessive accumulation of plasma macromolecules and decreased egress. Lipoproteins may then be irreversibly precipitated as atheromata in the composite plaque.

It should be emphasized that at the inception of atherosclerosis, intimal thickening represents the biologic response of blood vessels to the diminished wall pressure generated by the flowing blood at sites of predilection determined by the laws of fluid mechanics as they apply to local hydraulic specifications.

CURE VS. CONTROL OR MODIFICATION

Atherosclerosis is a progressive pathological process or disease. Apart from localized reaming procedures, bypass operations, and the replacement of surgically accessible diseased vessels, atherosclerosis, which affects all individuals in varying degrees, cannot be cured in the sense of curing or eliminating an infectious disease. Blood flow is necessary for life and blood flow inherently causes atherosclerotic changes in blood vessels. The best we can hope to achieve is to minimize or retard the development of atherosclerosis by controlling the relevant hydraulic specifications that control the development of atherosclerosis. It may be noted that not all the hydraulic factors that contribute to the development of atherosclerosis are of equal importance, nor are they all amenable to change, manipulation, or control. Thus, the anatomic patterns, such as angles of branching, radii of curvature, attachments, and calibers of lumens, are largely determined by heredity and development. Similarly, the biologic response of the intima to the stimulus of the hydraulic forces is probably determined by heredity as a racial or species characteristic.

A promising area of specific research lies in the study of the velocity of blood flow. An increase in blood velocity, if other factors remain unchanged, must produce more severe atherosclerosis (McAllister et al., 1960). A decrease in blood velocity, if achieved without impairing the metabolic requirements of vital centers or organs, may be expected to minimize or retard the development of atherosclerosis and its progressive pathological complications. A pharmacologic agent or a physiological method may be found or developed to achieve this goal.

Another valid research approach to the control of atherosclerosis lies in a study of methods to alter or modify the biologic factor, namely, the reactive reparative response of the intima or walls of blood vessels to the forces generated by the flowing blood.

CHARACTERISTICS OF BLOOD FLOW IN ARTERIES THAT INFLUENCE THE DEVELOPMENT OF ATHEROSCLEROSIS

In contrast to steady flow, which characteristically produces a relatively constant compressional or tensile stress at a given site in a blood vessel, pulsatile flow may be characterized by alternating compressional and tensile stresses. In pulsatile flow, a high mean velocity, a high peak velocity, and a high rate of change of velocity may be more prone to promote the development of intimal proliferation and atherosclerotic change than a lower average rate of flow, a lower peak velocity, and a lower rate of change of velocity. In this sense, a pulsatile flow that can be made to approach the characteristics of steady flow may be less prone to produce atherosclerosis.

Modifications of the features of pulsatile flow that may be expected to retard the development of atherosclerosis are: (1) a slower pulse rate, (2) a slower rate of change of blood velocity from minimum to maximum, (3) a decreased peak velocity, (4) a decreased mean velocity, and (5) a smaller range of blood velocity.

The velocity of blood flow is largely determined by the contractility of the myocardium (vis a tergo) and the peripheral resistance.

HYPERTENSION

In a general population, comparing those who remain free of clinical coronary disease and those who develop significant clinical disease, the analysis of blood pressure readings reveals there is no value, however large or small, that lies distinctly in the distribution of one group and not the other (Kannel, 1974). Simply stated, atherosclerosis is found in all individuals in varying grades of severity and without relation to the level of blood pressure in any individual case. It is notable that the precipitation of angina intentionally in the laboratory by exercise is followed by blood pressure elevation. However, the level of blood pressure prior to exercise is not of universal importance in the diagnosis or induction of angina pectoris (Riseman, 1936).

Theories that attempt to relate causally hypertension to atherosclerosis by degenerative changes in the intima due to vascularization (Paterson et al., 1960) or lipid filtration (Gofman and Young, 1963; Watts, 1963; Wilens, 1951) are flawed by the localization of atherosclerosis at zones of lower wall pressure rather than zones of higher wall pressure as determined by local blood flow patterns in the circulatory system.

Blood pressure studies that evaluate the clinical effect of therapy by diet, drugs, or life-style in relation to hypertension demonstrate no appreciable change in the natural course of coronary atherosclerosis as reflected in morbidity or mortality rates (Moyer, 1973; Veterans Study, 1970).

Nevertheless, the control of hypertension is to be encouraged in order to help prevent the complications of small vessel renal disease and of cerebral atherosclerotic vascular disease, particularly hemorrhage and stroke, while recognizing that vascular hemorrhage, including cerebral vascular hemorrhage, may occur in individuals with normal blood pressure due to their basic disease of atherosclerosis.

In summary it may be concluded that treatment for control of blood pressure is more effective in preventing stroke and congestive heart failure than in preventing the complications of coronary atherosclerosis. Coronary atherosclerosis and myocardial infarction occur in normotensive persons as well as in hypertensive persons. Hypertension may coexist as a complicating factor in coronary artery atherosclerosis without relation to the morbidity or mortality of coronary atherosclerosis. Atherosclerosis is basically due to the effect of the local velocity of blood flow and the local tensile force at the wall of the blood vessel rather than the level of systemic arterial pressure.

It is notable that the absolute pressure in a hydraulic system does not determine the velocity of flow. The velocity of flow is determined by a gradient—the difference in pressure between two points in a continuous system. If there is no difference in pressure between two points, there is no flow, regardless of the absolute pressure present. Thus, a reduction in the difference in pressure (gradient) will decrease the velocity flow between two points in a continuous hydraulic system. Locally, as well as generally, if these hydraulic conditions, namely, a decreased blood velocity and decreased gradient, can be achieved without impairing other metabolic requirements of the body, the development of atherosclerosis may be minimized or retarded.

EXERCISE

Exercise is a normal human activity and should be encouraged in order to maintain normal muscular tone and general physical fitness (Texon, 1976b). The types of physical exercise, the frequency, and duration of exercise periods must be adapted to each individual's requirements and physiological capacity. It should be emphasized again that atherosclerosis is a price we pay for blood flow and that an increase in blood velocity is uniformly the direct result of exercise. Furthermore, an increase in blood velocity produces vascular changes (intimal proliferation)—albeit on a microscopic scale but nevertheless in a cumulative manner (McAllister et al., 1960). This may be counteracted to some degree by athletic conditioning that slows the pulse and thus tends to modify the hydraulic characteristics of pulsatile flow (*vide supra*) in order to exert a minimum mechanical stress by diminishing the tensile stress upon the intima of blood vessels.

It should be noted that an individual with coronary arteries that are of large caliber with large radii of curvature can exercise with less risk of coronary occlusive atherosclerotic changes and clinical symptomatology at an early age than an individual who has coronary arteries with smaller diameters and sharper curvatures. Although exercise may reasonably be expected to improve general physical fitness, there is no scientific basis to indicate that coronary atherosclerosis is influenced beneficially by the increased blood velocity induced by exercise. It would clearly be unwise to advise a standard set of exercises for all individuals at any given age. Exercise should not be prescribed (Bruce and Kluge, 1971) to the stage of (1) excessive fatigue or exhaustion, (2) marked shortness of breath, or (3) chest pain. These symptoms are indicative of circulatory insufficiency. Healthy exertion or exercise should produce a "delicious fatigue," not exhaustion, acute dyspnea, or chest pain.

DIETARY FAT AND CHOLESTEROL

In 1965, the American Heart Association advised the general public to modify the fat and cholesterol of its diet in the hope that such dietary modification would lead to reduced levels of plasma cholesterol, retard the development of atherosclerosis, and reduce the incidence of all forms of atherosclerotic disease. The validity of this position as well as modified versions in 1973, 1975, and 1978, has been challenged (Stehbens, 1974, 1977; Mann, 1977) primarily because an unequivocal scientific demonstration that dietary control of hyperlipidemia reduces the mortality and morbidity of atherosclerotic disease is not presently available.

Despite continuing intensive epidemiological research (Kannel et al., 1971) and lipid research that has witnessed periodic shifting of emphasis (Ahrens, 1976) from total fat to cholesterol to saturated fat to unsaturated fat to triglycerides and most recently to low-density lipoproteins and high-density lipoproteins, there is as yet no unequivocal evidence that reduction of lipid levels or any of its fractions by diet or drugs influences the pathological process or lowers the risk of any form of atherosclerotic disease. The most recent review of the Framington

Study states that the previous position, that virtually all of the lipid information pertaining to coronary heart disease resided in the serum total cholesterol, must be modified (Kannel et al., 1979).

Studies that raise serum cholesterol by increasing dietary cholesterol and fat intake leading to atherosclerotic lesions in animals (Antischkow, 1913, 1933, 1967; Taylor et al., 1963) and regression of the lesions by cessation of those diets (Armstrong, 1976; Armstrong et al., 1970; Fritz et al., 1976; Vesselinovitch et al., 1976; Wissler, 1978) are flawed. They are flawed by the high levels of lipidemia required that lead to excessive overloading or fat storage in almost all the potential fat depots of the tissues and organs of the body. There is no correlation between blood cholesterol levels and the severity of atherosclerotic vascular disease in the general population (Garrett et al., 1964, Page, 1977; Talbott, 1961). Nor is there any relation between the daily nutritional intake and serum lipid levels in a total community (Nichols et al., 1976). Atherosclerosis, including coronary atherosclerosis and myocardial infarction, occurs without relation in a causative sense (Stehbens, 1975b) to the level of cholesterol or any lipid fraction in the blood. The statement by Anitschkow (1933) that atherosclerotic changes in the rabbit are not found unless cholesterol is fed has been refuted by the finding of atherosclerotic changes in normal rabbits (Bragdon, 1952; Haust and More, 1965; Schenk, 1966a, 1966b; More, 1973).

After spending many years studying the production of atherosclerosis in animals by the maintenance of high serum cholesterol levels, Kendall (1967) concluded that it is extremely unlikely that the cholesterol content of the diet is more than a minor factor in the pathogenesis of human atherosclerosis. He pointed out that atherosclerotic lesions also occur in individuals with low serum lipid levels. He stated that the initial step in the process is damage to the cells of the arterial wall, and he suggested that it is futile to attempt to modify the incidence of atherosclerosis in a population by measures aimed primarily at lowering serum lipid levels without at the same time correcting the physiological factors that are causing the initial damage to the arterial walls.

To find fat in an atherosclerotic plaque when examined under the microscope and therefore to conclude that fat is the cause or contributes causally to plaque formation is, in my opinion, contrary to logical thinking and scientific facts. An analogous error would be to claim that leukocytes in an abscess are the cause of the abscess and an individual with fewer leukocytes would have a lesser pathological response. Obviously, the cause of an abscess is a noxious stimulus, for example, bacterial infection, and the biologic response is the local leukocytic reaction. Similarly, fat droplets and cholesterol crystals found in atherosclerotic plaques are part of the pathological *in situ* response to vascular injury arising from the forces (diminished wall pressure) generated by the flowing blood at the specific sites of predilection in the circulatory system in accordance with the laws of fluid mechanics. Examples of fatty change are not uncommon in the body as a result of toxic or noxious agents, for example, alcoholic fatty change in the liver, fatty change associated with thyroid hemorrhagic pathology, lipid deposition in interstitial pneumonitis (Waddell et al., 1954a), and lipids in the inflammatory response in lung and muscle (Waddell et al., 1954b).

SUMMARY

The development of atherosclerosis is a sequel to the forces of blood flow and is found in varying degrees of severity in all individuals at sites of predilection in the circulatory system characterized by diminished lateral pressure in accordance with the effects of the laws of fluid mechanics (Texon, 1957; Texon et al., 1962, 1965). The effect of the laws of fluid mechanics is the primary causative or etiologic factor for the development of atherosclerosis (Texon, 1960a, 1960b). Atherosclerosis may be considered the reactive biologic response of the arteries to the forces generated by the flowing blood.

It is notable that within physiological limits, a slower pulse rate, a lower average blood velocity, a lower peak velocity, a lower rate of change in velocity, a decrease in peak contractility of the heart, and a decrease in pulse pressure are hydraulic conditions that may be expected to minimize or retard the development of atherosclerosis.

Pulsatile flow, as found in the circulatory system, is characterized by hydraulic features and specifications that are more conducive to the production of atherosclerosis than steady flow.

The reparative response of the intima at the cellular level to the forces of flowing blood (the biologic factor) should be further explored as another valid approach to control of the atherosclerotic process.

Atherosclerosis cannot be cured in the sense of curing an infectious disease. We may look forward to the control or modification of blood velocity and other relevant hydraulic factors that cause atherosclerosis (Texon, 1973, 1974). We may then retard the rate of development of atherosclerotic vascular disease and consequently extend the human life span.

REFERENCES

Ahrens EH Jr: The management of hyperlipidemia: Whether, rather than how. Ann Intern Med 85:87-93, 1976.

Altschul R: Endothelium, Its Development, Morphology, Function and Pathology. New York: Macmillan, 1954.

Altschule MD, editor: Med Clin North Am—Symposium on Atherosclerosis. Philadelphia: Saunders, 1974.

Anitschkow N: Uber die veranderungen der kaninchenaorto bei experimenteller cholesteatose. Beitr Pathol 56:379, 1913.

Anitschkow N: Experimental arteriosclerosis in animals. In: Arteriosclerosis—A Survey of the Problem, edited by EV Cowdry, pp. 271-322. New York: Macmillan, 1933.

Anitschkow N: A history of experimentation on arterial atherosclerosis in animals, Cowdry's arteriosclerosis (2nd edition), edited by HT Blumenthal, pp. 21-44, Springfield, Ill.: Thomas, 1967.

Anliker M, Maxwell JA: The dispersion of waves in blood vessels. In: Symposium on Biomechanics. New York: Appl Mech Div of ASME, 1966.

Armstrong ML: Regression of atherosclerosis. In: Atherosclerosis, edited by R Paoletti, AM Gotto Jr., vol. 1, pp. 131-182. New York: Raven Press, 1976.

Armstrong ML, Warner ED, Connor WE: Regression of coronary atheromatosis in rhesus monkeys. Circ Res 27:59-67, 1970.

Astrup P, Kjeldsen K: Carbon monoxide, smoking, and atherosclerosis. In: Med Clin North Am—Symposium on Atherosclerosis, edited by MD Altschule, 58:332-350. Philadelphia: Saunders, 1974.

Attinger EO, editor: Pulsatile Blood Flow. New York: McGraw-Hill, 1964.

Balint A: The fine structure of the mammalian arterial wall. In: Arterial Lesions and Arteriosclerosis, edited by H Jellinek, Budapest: Akademiai Kiado, 1974.

Baumann FG, Imparato AM, Kim G: The evolution of early fibromuscular lesions hemodynamically induced in the dog renal artery. Circ Res 39:809-827, 1976.

Benditt EP, Benditt JM: Evidence for a monoclonal origin of human atherosclerotic plaques. Proc Natl Acad Sci USA 70:1753-1756, 1973.

Bergel DH: The static elastic properties of the arterial wall. J. Physiol 156:445-457, 1961.

Billings FT Jr: Variability of serum cholesterol in hypercholesterolemia. Arch Intern Med 110:53-56, 1962.

Binder RC: Fluid Mechanics. Englewood Cliffs, N.J.: Prentice-Hall, 1955.

Bjorkerus S, Bondjers G: Endothelial integrity and velocity in the aorta of the normal rabbit and not as evaluated with dye exclusion tests and interference contrast microscopy. Atherosclerosis 15:285-300, 1972.

Bragdon JH: Spontaneous atherosclerosis in the rabbit. Circulation 5:641, 1952.

Bruce RA, Kluge W: Defibrillatory treatment of exertional cardiac arrest in coronary disease: Possible lethal peril of violent exercise to coronary artery disease patients. JAMA 216:613-658, 1971.

Bugliarello G: Microcirculation hemodynamics and other biological flow problems. In: Biomedical Fluid Mechanics Symposium. New York: Fluids Engineering Div, ASME, pp. 192-208, 1966.

Burchell, HB: Aortic dissection. Circulation 12:1068, 1955.

Burchell HB: Editorial. Heart attacks and Workmen's Compensation Acts, Circulation 33:345, 1966.

Caro CG: Transport of material between blood and wall in arteries. Ciba Found Symp 12:127-148, 1973.

Caro CG, Fitz-Gerald JM, Schroter RC: Atheroma and arterial wall shear: Observation, correlation and proposal of shear dependent mass transfer mechanisms for atherogenesis. Proc R Soc Lond 177:109-159, 1971.

Chapman JM, Massey FJ: The interrelationship of serum cholesterol, hypertension, body weight, and risk of coronary disease: Results of the first ten years' follow-up in the Los Angeles Heart Study. J Chronic Dis 17:933-949, 1964.

Chernick S, Spere PA, Chaikoff IL: The metabolism of arterial tissue. J Biol Chem 179:113, 1949.

Cohen MI: Analysis and measurement of fluid flow in distensible tubes, with application of blood flow in arteries. Doctoral Thesis. Troy, NY: Rensselaer Polytechnic, 1964.

Corday E, Corday SR: Prevention of heart disease by control of risk factors: The time has come to face the facts. Am J Cardiol 35:330-333, 1975.

Davids N, Cheng RC: Finite element analysis of flow in blood vessel with arbitrary cross-section. NIH Progress Report, Dept of Engineering Mechanics, Pennsylvania State Univ, January, 1972.

Davids N, Cheng RC, Melville JG: Laminar pulsatile flow problems by finite element analysis methods. Proceedings, 3rd Canadian Congress of Applied Mechanics, pp. 789-790. Alberta, Canada, 1971.

Duguid JB, Robertson WB: Mechanical factors in atherosclerosis. Lancet 1:1205-1209, 1957.

Ergatoudis I, Irons BM, Zienkiewics DC: Curved isoparametric quadrilateral elements for finite element analysis. Int J Solids Struct 4:31-42, 1968.

Evans, RL: Pulsatile flow in vessels whose distensibility and size vary with site. Phys Med Biol 7:105-116, 1962.

Fishman JA, Ryan GB, Karnovsky MJ: Endothelial regeneration in the rat carotid artery and the significance of endothelial denudation in the pathogenesis of myointimal thickening. Lab Invest 32:339–351, 1975.

Fredrickson DS, Levy RI, Lees RS: Fat transport in lipoproteins: An integrated approach to mechanisms and disorders. N Engl J Med 276:34–44, 94–103, 148–156, 215–225, 273–281, 1967.

French JE: Atherosclerosis in relation to the structure and function of the arterial intima, with special reference to the endothelium. Int Rev Exp Pathol 5:253–353, 1966.

Friedman M, and Rosenman RH: Type A Behavior and Your Heart. New York: Knopf, 1974.

Friedman M, Manwaring JH, Rosenman RH, Dohlon G, Ortega P, Grube SM: Instantaneous and sudden deaths, clinical and pathological differentiation in coronary artery disease, JAMA 225:1319–1328, 1973.

Friedman RJ, Moore S, Singal DP: Repeated endothelial injury and induction of atherosclerosis in normolipemic rabbits by human serum. Lab Invest 32:404–415, 1975.

Fritz KE, Augustyn JM, Jarmolych J, Daoud AS, Lee KY: Regression of advanced atherosclerosis in swine. Arch Pathol 100:380–385, 1976.

Fry DL: Acute vascular endothelial changes associated with increased blood velocity gradients. Circ Res 22:165–197, 1968.

Fry DL: Certain chemorheologic considerations regarding the blood vascular interface with particular reference to coronary artery disease. Circulation 39–40 (suppl 4):4–38, 1969.

Fry DL: Responses of the arterial wall to certain physical factors. Ciba Found Symp 12:93–125, 1973.

Fry DL, Noble FW, Mallos AJ: An electric device for instantaneous computation of aortic blood velocity. Circ Res 5:75–78, 1957.

Gabe IT: An analogue computer deriving oscillatory arterial blood flow from the pressure gradient. Phys Med Biol 10:407–415, 1965.

Garrett HE, Horning EC, Creech BG, DeBakey M: Serum cholesterol levels in patients treated surgically for atherosclerosis. JAMA 189:655–659, 1964.

Geer JC, Haust MD: Smooth muscle cells in atherosclerosis. In: Monographs on atherosclerosis, edited by OJ Pollack, HS Simms, and JE Kirk, vol 2, pp. 1–88, Basel: Karger, 1972.

Gessner FB: Hemodynamic theories of atherogenesis. Circ Res 33:259–266, 1973.

Glagov S: Hemodynamic risk factors: Mechanical stress, mural architecture, medial nutrition and the vulnerability of arteries to atherosclerosis. In: The Pathogenesis of Atherosclerosis, edited by JC Geer, pp. 164–199. Baltimore: Williams & Wilkins, 1972.

Gofman JW, Young W: The filtration concept of atherosclerosis and serum lipids in the diagnosis of atherosclerosis. In: Atherosclerosis and Its Origin, edited by M Sandler, GH Bourne, pp. 197–229. New York: Academic Press, 1963.

Gutstein WH, Schneck DJ, Marks JO: In vitro studies of local blood flow disturbances in a region of separation. J Atherosclerosis Res 8:381–388, 1968.

Gyurko G, Szabo M: Experimental investigations of the role of hemodynamic factors in formation of intimal changes. Surgery 66:871–874, 1969.

Haust MD: Arterial endothelium and its potentials. In: Atherosclerosis, Metabolic, Morphologic and Clinical Aspects, edited by GW Manning, MD Haust, pp. 34-49. New York: Plenum Press, 1976.

Haust MD, More RH: Spontaneous lesions of the aorta in the rabbit. In: Comparative Atherosclerosis, p. 255. New York: Hoeber, 1965.

Haust MD, More RH, Movat HZ: The mechanism of fibrosis in arteriosclerosis. Am J Pathol 35:265, 1959.

Hollander W: Role of hypertension in atherosclerosis and cardiovascular disease. Am J Cardiol 38:786-800, 1976.

Hung TK, Naff SA: A mathematical model of systolic blood flow through a bifurcation. In: Eighth International Conference on Medical and Biological Engineering. Chicago, 1969.

Imparato AM, Lord JW, Texon M, Helpern M: Experimental atherosclerosis produced by alteration of blood vessel configuration. Surg Forum, 12:245, 1961.

Imparato AM, Baumann FG, Pearson J, Kim GE, Davidson T, Ibrahim I, Nathan I: Electron microscopic studies of experimentally produced fibromuscular lesions. Surg Gynecol Obstet 139:497-504, 1974.

Jellinek H, editor: Arterial Lesions and Arteriosclerosis. Budapest: Akademiai Kiado, 1974.

Jenkins CD: Psychologic and social precursors of coronary disease: N Engl J Med 284:244-255, 307-317, 1971.

Kannel WB: The role of cholesterol in coronary atherosclerosis. In: Med Clin North Am—Symposium on Atherosclerosis, edited by MD Altschule, 58:363-379, Philadelphia: Saunders, 1974.

Kannel WB, Gordon T: The Framingham study: An epidemiological investigation of cardiovascular diseases. In: Section 24, Diet and the regulation of serum cholesterol, edited by WB Kannel, T Gordon. US Department of Health, Education and Welfare, Public Health Service, National Institutes of Health (No. 1740-0329). Washington, DC: Government Printing Office, 1971.

Kannel WB, Castelli WP, Gordon T: Cholesterol in the prediction of atherosclerotic disease. Ann Intern Med 90:85-91, 1979.

Kannel WB, Castelli WP, Gordon T, McNamara PM: Serum cholesterol, lipoproteins, and the risk of coronary heart disease. Ann Intern Med 74:1-12, 1971.

Kannel WB, Dawber TR, Sorlie P, Wolf PA: Components of blood pressure and risk of atherothrombotic brain infarction: The Framingham study. Stroke 7:327-331, 1976.

Kendall FE: Editorial. Does the pattern of carbohydrate metabolism hold a clue to atherosclerosis? Circulation 36:340-344, 1967.

Kern WH, Dermer GB, Lindesmith GG: The intimal proliferation in aortic-coronary saphenous vein grafts. Am Heart J 84:771-777, 1972.

Keys A, editor: Coronary heart disease in seven countries. Circulation 41 (suppl 1): I1-I211, 1970.

Krovetz LJ: The effect of vessel branching on haemodynamic stability. Phys Med Biol 10 (No. 3): 417-427, 1965.

Lynn NS, Fox VG, Ross LW: Flow patterns at arterial bifurcations. In: Symposium Am Inst Ch Eng, 63rd Annual Meeting Chicago, 1970.

Mann GV: Diet-heart: End of an era. New Eng J Med 297:644-650, 1977.

McAllister FF, Bertsch R, Jacobson J, II, D'Allesio G: The accelerating effect of muscular exercise on experimental atherosclerosis. Arch Surg. 80:54-60, 1960.

McConalogue DJ, Srivastava RS: Motion of a fluid in a curved tube. Proc R Soc London 307:37, 1968.

McDonald DA: Blood Flow in Arteries. Baltimore: Williams & Wilkins, 1974.

McMichael J: Prevention of coronary heart disease. Lancet 2:569, 1976.

Mitchell JRA, Schwartz CJ: Arterial Disease. Oxford: Blackwell, 1965.

More S: Thromboatherosclerosis in normolipemic rabbits: A result of continued endothelial damage. Lab Invest 29:478, 1973.

Moser M, Goldman AG: Hypertensive Vascular Disease. Philadelphia: Lippincott, 1967.

Moyer JH, Flynn J: The role of arterial hypertension in coronary atherosclerosis. In: Coronary Heart Disease, edited by HI Russek, BL Zohman, pp. 137-145. Philadelphia: Lippincott, 1971.

Moyer, JH: Frequency, adequacy and significance of therapy for arterial hypertension in the United States today. In: Major Advances in Cardiovascular Therapy, edited by HI Russek, pp. 285-294. Baltimore: Williams & Wilkins, 1973.

Mustard JF, Packham MA: Factors influencing platelet function: Adhesion, release, and aggregation. Pharmacol Rev 22:97-187, 1970.

Mustard JF, Packham MA: The role of blood and platelets in atherosclerosis and the complications of atherosclerosis. Thromb Diath Haemorrh 33:444-456, 1975.

Nichols AB, Ravenscroft C, Lamphiear DE, Ostrander DE: Daily nutritional intake and serum lipid levels: The Tecumseh study. Am J Clin Nutr 29:1384-1392, 1976.

Noordergraaf A, Verdouw PD, van Brummelen AGW, Wiegel FW: Analog of the arterial bed. In: Pulsatile Blood Flow, edited by EO Attinger, pp. 373-387. New York: McGraw-Hill, 1964.

Oberman A, et al.: The cardiovascular risk: Associated with different levels and types of elevated blood pressure. Minn Med 52:1283-1288, 1969.

Ogden E: An experimental study of induced pulse waves in arteries. Atlantic City, Fed Proc, 1966.

Page IH: The Cholesterol Fallacy. Cleveland: Coronary Club, 1977.

Patel DJ, Greenfield JC Jr, Fry DL: In vivo pressure-length-radius relationship of certain blood vessels in man and dog. In: Pulsatile Blood Flow, edited by AO Attinger, pp. 293-305. New York: McGraw-Hill, 1964.

Paterson JC, Hill J, Lockwood CH: The role of hypertension in the progression of atherosclerosis. Can Med Assoc J 82:65, 1960.

Pedley TJ, Schroter RC, Sudlow MF: Flow and pressure drop in systems of repeatedly branching tubes. J Fluid Mechanics 46:365-383, 1971.

Pickering G: Hypertension (2nd edition). New York: Longman, 1974.

Reemtsma K, Sandberg LB, Greenfield NN: Some theoretic aspects of vascular degeneration. Am J Surg 119:548-552, 1970.

Report of the Committee on the Effect of Strain and Trauma on the Heart and Blood Vessels. Circulation 26:612, 1962.

Rindfleisch E: A Textbook of Pathologic Histology, translated by WC Kloman and FT Miles, pp. 211-212. Philadelphia: Lindsay-Blakiston, 1872.

Riseman JEF: The relation of the systolic blood pressure and heart rate to attacks of angina pectoris precipitated by effort. Am Heart J 12:53, 1936.

Roberts WC, Bujo LM: The frequency and significance of coronary arterial thrombi and other observations in fatal acute myocardial infarction. Am J Med 52:425-443, 1972.

Roberts WC, Levy RI, Fredrickson DS: Hyperlipoproteinemia. Arch Pathol 90:46-56, 1970.

Roberts WC, Ferrans VJ, Levy RI, Fredrickson DS: Cardiovascular pathology in hyperlipoproteinemia. Am J Cardiol 31:557-570, 1973.

Robertson TL, Kato H, Gordon T, et al.: Epidemiologic studies of coronary heart disease and stroke in Japanese men living in Japan, Hawaii and California: Coronary heart disease risk factors in Japan and Hawaii. Am J Cardiol 39:244-249, 1977a.

Robertson TL, Kato H, Rhoads GG, et al.: Epidemiologic studies of coronary heart disease and stroke in Japanese men living in Japan, Hawaii and California: Incidence of myocardial infarction and death from coronary heart disease. Am J Cardiol 39:239-243, 1977b.

Rodkiewicz CM, Roussel CL: Fluid mechanics in a large arterial bifurcation. Trans ASME, J Fluids Eng, 72-WA/FE-8, 108, March 1973.

Rosenman RH, Friedman M: The possible role of behavior patterns in proneness and immunity to coronary heart disease. In: Coronary Heart Disease, edited by HI Russek, BL Zohman, pp. 74-84. Philadelphia: Lippincott, 1971.

Rosenman RH, Friedman M: Neurogenic factors in pathogenesis of coronary heart disease. In: Med Clin North Am—Symposium on Atherosclerosis, edited by MD Altschule. Philadelphia: Saunders, 1974.

Ross, R, Glomset JA: Atherosclerosis and the arterial smooth muscle cell. Science 180:1332-1339, 1973.

Rubinow SI, Keller JB: Theoretical aspects of blood flow in arteries. In: Proc First International Conf on Hemorheology. Oxford: Pergamon Press, 1966.

Rudinger G: Review of current mathematical methods for the analysis of blood flow. In: Biomedical Fluid Mechanics Symposium. New York: ASME Fluids Engineering Div, pp. 1-33, April 1966.

Rushmer RF: Cardiovascular Dynamics. Philadelphia: Saunders, 1970.

Russek HI: Role of emotional stress in atherosclerosis. In: Atherosclerotic Vascular Disease, edited by AN Brest, JH Moyer, pp. 106-114. New York: Appleton-Century-Crofts, 1967.

Schenk EA, Gaman E, Feigenbaum AS: Spontaneous aortic lesions in rabbits—morphologic characteristics. Circ Res 19:80-88, 1966a.

Schenk EA, Gaman E, Feigenbaum AS: Spontaneous aortic lesions in rabbits—relationship to experimental atherosclerosis. Circ Res 19:89-95, 1966b.

Schneck DJ, Gutstein WH: Boundary layer studies in blood flow. In: ASME Publication No. 66—WA (BHF-4, 1966).

Schroeder HA: The role of trace elements in cardiovascular disease. In: Med Clin North Am 58:381-396, Philadelphia: Saunders, 1974.

Schultz DL: Pressure and flow in large arteries. In: Cardiovascular Fluid Dynamics, edited by DH Bergel, vol. 1, p. 291. New York: Academic Press, 1972.

Skalak R, Stathis T: A porous tapered elastic tube model of a vascular bed.

In: Symposium on Biomechanics. New York: Appl Mech Div of ASME, 1966.

Skalak R, Zarda PR, Chen PH, Chen TC: A variational principle for slow viscous flow with suspended particles. In: Study No. 5, Computer-Aided Engineering. Waterloo, Canada: University of Waterloo, 1970.

Smith EB, Alexander KM, Massie IB. Quantitative studies of the interaction between plasma and tissue components in human intima. In: Atherosclerosis, Metabolic, Morphologic and Clinical Aspects, edited by GW Manning, MD Haust, pp. 872–877. New York: Plenum Press, 1976.

Spaet TH, Gaynor E, Stemerman MB: Thrombosis, atherosclerosis, and endothelium. Am Heart J 87:661–667, 1974.

Stamler J, Lindberg HA, Berkson DM, et al. Prevalence and incidence of coronary heart disease in strata of the labor force of a Chicago industrial corporation. J Chronic Dis 11:405–420, 1960.

Stehbens WE: Turbulence of blood flow in the vascular system of man. In: Flow Properties of Man, edited by AL Copley, G Stainsby. New York: Pergamon Press, 1960.

Stehbens WE: Blood vessel changes in chronic experimental arteriovenous fistulas. Surg Gynecol Obstet 127:327, 1968.

Stehbens WE: Haemodynamic production of lipid deposition, intimal tears, mural dissection and thrombosis in the blood vessel wall. Proc R Soc London (Biol) 185:357–373, 1974.

Stehbens WE: Flow in glass models of arterial bifurcations and berry aneurysms at low Reynolds numbers. QJ Exp Physiol 60:181–192, 1975a.

Stehbens WE: The role of lipid in the pathogenesis of atherosclerosis. Lancet 1:724–727, 1975b.

Stehbens WE: The interrelation of hypertension, lipid, and atherosclerosis. Cardiovasc Med 2:263–277, 1977.

Stehbens WE, Karmody AM: Venous atherosclerosis associated with arteriovenous fistulas for hemodialysis. Arch Surg 110:176–180, 1975.

Streeter VL, Keitzer WF, Bohr FF: Pulsatile pressure and flow through distensible vessels. Circ Res 13:3–20, 1963.

Talbott GD: Limitations of serum cholesterol level as diagnostic index of cardiovascular status. J Am Geriatr Soc 9:825–832, 1961.

Taylor CB, Patton DE, Cox GE: Atherosclerosis in rhesus monkeys. VI. Fatal myocardial infarction in a monkey fed fat and cholesterol. Arch Pathol 76:404–412, 1963.

Texon M: Heart Disease and Industry. New York: Grune & Stratton, 1954.

Texon M: A hemodynamic concept of atherosclerosis with particular reference to coronary occlusion. AMA Arch Intern Med 99:418, 1957.

Texon M: Causal relationships in heart disease in workmen's compensation cases. In: Work and the Heart, edited by FF Rosenbaum and EL Belknap. New York: Hoeber, 1959.

Texon M: The hemodynamic concept of atherosclerosis. Bull NY Acad Med 36:263, 1960a.

Texon M: The hemodynamic concept of atherosclerosis (Editorial). Am J Cardiol 5:291, 1960b.

Texon M: The role of vascular hemodynamics in the development of atherosclerosis. In: Atherosclerosis and Its Origin, edited by M Sandler, GH Bourne. New York: Academic Press, 1963.

Texon M: Mechanical factors involved in atherosclerosis. In: Atherosclerotic Vascular Disease, edited by AN Brest, JH Moyer. New York: Appleton-Century-Crofts, 1967.

Texon M: The role of vascular dynamics (mechanical factors) in the development of atherosclerosis. In: Coronary Heart Disease, edited by HI Russek. Philadelphia: Lippincott Co. 1971.

Texon M: The hemodynamic basis of atherosclerosis. Further observations: the ostial lesion. Bull NY Acad Med 48:733–740, 1972.

Texon M: Vascular dynamics and the prevention of coronary heart disease. In: The Paul D. White Symposium: Major Advances in Cardiovascular Therapy, edited by HI Russek. Baltimore: Williams & Wilkins, 1973.

Texon M: Atherosclerosis—Its hemodynamic basis and implications. In: Med Clin North Am Symposium on Atherosclerosis, edited by MD Altschule. Philadelphia: Saunders, 1974.

Texon M: The hemodynamic basis of atherosclerosis. Further observations: The bifurcation lesion. Bull NY Acad Med 52:187–200, 1976a.

Texon M: The hemodynamic basis of atherosclerosis with special reference to physical exercise. In: Advances in Cardiology, vol. 18, pp. 122–135, Basel: Karger, 1976b.

Texon M, Imparato AM, Lord JW: Hemodynamic concept of atherosclerosis—Experimental production of arterial wall lesions. AMA Arch Surg 80:47, 1960.

Texon M, Imparato AM, Lord JW, Helpern M: The experimental production of arterial lesions furthering the hemodynamic concept of atherosclerosis. AMA Arch Intern Med 110:50, 1962.

Texon M, Imparato AM, Helpern M: The role of vascular dynamics in the development of atherosclerosis. JAMA 194:1226, 1965.

Thomas WA, Jones R, Scott RF, et al.: Production of early atherosclerotic lesions in rats characterized by proliferation of "modified smooth muscle cells." Exp Mol Pathol 1 (Suppl 2):40–61, 1963.

Tillotson JL, Kato H, Nichaman MZ, et al: Epidemiology of coronary heart disease and stroke in Japanese men living in Japan, Hawaii, and California: Methodology for comparison of diet. Am J Clin Nutr 26:177–184, 1973.

Veress B, Kadar A, Jellinek H: Ultra-structural elements in experimental intimal thickening. Exp Mol Pathol, 1969.

Vesselinovitch D, Wissler RW, Hughes R, et al: Reversal of advanced atherosclerosis in rhesus monkeys. Atherosclerosis 23:155–176, 1976.

Veterans Administration cooperative study group on antihypertensive agents: Effects of treatment on morbidity in hypertension. J Am Med Assoc 213:1143, 1970.

Waddell WR, Sniffen RC, Whytehead LL: The etiology of chronic interstitial pneumonitis associated with lipid deposition. J Thorac Cardiovasc Surg 28:134–144, 1954a.

Waddell WR, Sniffen RC, Whytehead LL: Influence of blood lipid levels on inflammatory response in lung and muscle. Am J Pathol 30:757–769, 1954b.

Watts HF: The mechanism of arterial lipid accumulation in human coronary artery atherosclerosis. In: Coronary Heart Disease, edited by W Likoff, JH Moyer, p. 98. New York: Grune & Stratton, 1963.

Werko L: Risk factors and coronary heart disease—Facts or fancy? Am Heart J 91:87–98, 1976.

Wiener F, Morkin E, Skalak R, Fishman AP: Wave propagation in the pulmonary circulation. Circ Res 19: 834, 1966.

Wilens SL: The experimental production of lipid deposition in excised arteries. Science 114:389, 1951.

Wissler RW: The arterial medial cell, smooth muscle or multifunctional mesenchyma. Circulation 36:1, 1967.

Wissler RW: Development of the atherosclerotic plaque. In: The Myocardium: Failure and Infarction, edited by E. Braunwald, pp. 155-166. New York: HP Publishing Company, 1974.

Wissler RW: Risk Factors and Regression in Atherosclerosis—Is It Reversible?, edited by G Schettler, E Stange, RW Wissler. New York: Springer-Verlag, 1978.

Wissler RW, Geer JC, editors: The Pathogenesis of Atherosclerosis. Baltimore: Williams & Wilkins, 1972.

Wormersley JR: An elastic tube theory of pulse transmission and oscillatory flow in mammalian arteries. In: Wright Air Development Center, WADC Report TR 56-614, 1957.

Wylie EB: Flow through tapered tubes with nonlinear wall properties. In: Symposium on Biomechanics. New York: Appl Mech Div of ASME, 1966.

Yudkin J: Diet and coronary thrombosis: Hypothesis and fact. Lancet 2:155-162, 1957.

Zemplenyi T: Vascular enzymes and the relevance of their study to problems of atherogenesis. In: Med Clin North Am—Symposium on Atherosclerosis, edited by MD Altschule 58:293-321. Philadelphia: Saunders, 1974.

Zemplenyi T, Lojda Z, Mrhova O: Enzymes of the vascular wall in experimental atherosclerosis in the rabbit. In: Atherosclerosis and Its Origin, edited by M Sandler, GH Bourne. New York: Academic Press, 1963.

BIBLIOGRAPHY

Altschul R: Selected Studies on Arteriosclerosis. Springfield, Ill.: Thomas, 1950.

American Heart Assoc: Comm on Nutrition, Diet and Coronary Heart Disease, New York: AHA, 1965.

American Heart Assoc: Comm on Nutrition, Diet and Coronary Heart Disease, New York: AHA, 1973.

American Heart Assoc Committee Report: On value and safety of diet modification to control hyperlipidemia in childhood and adolescence. Circulation 58:381A–385A, 1978.

Baker AB, Resch JA, Loewenson RB: Hypertension and cerebral atherosclerosis. Circulation 39:701–710, 1969.

Benditt EP: The origin of atherosclerosis. Sci Am 236(2):74–85, 1977.

Brill IC, Brodeur MTH, Oyama AA: Myocardial infarction in two sisters less than 20 years old. JAMA 217(10): 1345–1348, 1971.

Brown MS, Faust JR, Goldstein JL: Role of the low density lipoprotein receptor in regulating the content of free and esterified cholesterol in human fibroblasts. J Clin Invest 55:783–793, 1975.

Burton AC: Physiology and Biophysics of the Circulation. Chicago: Year Book Medical Publishers, 1965.

Caro CG, Pedley TJ, Schroter RC, Seed, WA: The Mechanics of the Circulation. New York: Oxford University Press, 1978.

Cholesterol Metabolism (Editorial), Lancet 2:524–525, 1973.

Coronary Drug Project Research Group: The coronary drug project: Initial findings leading to modifications of its research protocol. JAMA 214:1303–1313, 1970.

Coronary Drug Project Research Group: The coronary drug project: Findings leading to further modifications of its protocol with respect to dexrothyroxine. JAMA 220:996–1008, 1972.

Coronary Drug Project Research Group: The coronary drug project: Design methods and baseline results. Circulation 47 (suppl 1): I1-I150, 1973.

Coronary Drug Project Research Group: Clofibrate and niacin in coronary heart disease. JAMA 231:360–381, 1975.

Daily JW, Hareman DRF: Fluid Dynamics. Reading, Mass.: Addison Wesley, 1966.

Durand WF: The outlook in fluid mechanics. Journal of the Franklin Institute 228:183, 1939.

Epstein FJ, Ostrander LD, Johnson BC: Epidemiological studies of cardiovascular disease in a total community—Tecumseh, Michigan. Ann Intern Med 62:1170–1187, 1965.

Fishman AP, Richards DW, editors: Circulation of Blood: Men and Ideas. New York: Oxford University Press, 1964.

Frantz ID: The rationale for hypolipemic therapy. Handbook Exp Pharmacol 41:409–415, 1975.

Fraser R: The limitations of statistical correlations in pathology. Pathology 7:113–116, 1975.

Frasher WG: What is known about the physiology of large blood vessels. In: Colloquium on Biomechanics. Applied Mech Div of the ASME, 1966.

Fry DL: Certain histological and chemical responses of the vascular interface to acutely induced mechanical stress in the aorta of the dog. Circulation Res 24:93, 1969.

Goldstein JL, Brown MS: Binding and degradation of low density lipoproteins by cultured human fibroblasts: Comparison of cells from a normal subject and from a patient with homozygous familial hypercholesterolemia. J Biol Chem 249:5153–5162, 1974.

Gordon T, Kannel WB: Predisposition to atherosclerosis in the head, heart and legs—The Framingham study. JAMA 221:66, 1972.

Gordon T, Kannel WB, editors: The Framingham study. National Heart and Lung Institute, Monograph Sections 1–26, Bethesda, 1968–70.

Gordon T, Kannel WB, Sorlie PD: The Framingham study: 16-year follow-up, Washington, DC: DHEW, 1971.

Herem RM, Cornhill JF: The role of fluid mechanics in atherogenesis. Proceedings from National Science Foundation Meeting, The Ohio State University, Columbus, August 24–25, 1978

Heyman A, Nefzger MD, Estes EH Jr: Serum cholesterol level in cerebral infarction, Arch Neurol 5:264–268, 1961.

Laragh JH: Renal and adrenal factors in hypertension: Diagnostic approaches. Bull NY Acad Med 45:859–876, 1969.

Lyne WH: Unsteady flow in a curved pipe. J Fluid Mechanics 45:13, 1971.

The Masai's cholesterol. Editorial: Br Med J 3:262–263, 1971.

McGill HC Jr editor: Geographic Pathology of Atherosclerosis. Baltimore: Williams & Wilkins, 1968.

McMichael J: Fats and atheroma: An inquest. Br Med J 1:173–175, 1979.

Mustard JF, Rowsell HC, Murphy EA, Downie HG: Evolution of the Atherosclerotic Plaque, edited by RJ Jones. Chicago: University of Chicago Press, 1963.

National Heart, Lung, and Blood Institute (Fourth Report of the): National Heart, Blood Vessel, Lung, and Blood Program. (DHEW Publication No. (NIH) 77-1170). Bethesda, Md: Public Health Service, National Institutes of Health, 1977.

Primary prevention of the atherosclerotic diseases: Inter-Society Commission for Heart Disease Resources. Circulation 42:A55–A95, 1970.

Ross R: The arterial smooth muscle cell. In: The Pathogenesis of Atherosclerosis, edited by RW Wissler, JC Geer, pp. 147–163. Baltimore: Williams & Wilkins, 1972.

Ross R., Glomset J: Studies of primate arterial smooth muscle cells in relation to atherosclerosis. Arterial Mesenchyme and Arteriosclerosis, edited by WD Wagner, TB Clarkson, pp. 265–279. New York: Plenum Press, 1974.

Ross R, Harker L: Hyperlipidemia and atherosclerosis. Science 193:1094–1099, 1976.

Scarton HA, Shah PM, Tsapogas MJ: The role of hemodynamics in early atheroma in the aorta. In: Biomechanics Symposium Proceedings, ASME Summer Applied Mechanics Conference, June 23–25, pp. 15–16, Troy, N.Y.: Rensselaer Polytechnic Institute, 1975.

Schlichting H: Boundary-Layer Theory. New York: McGraw-Hill, 1955.

Schwartz SM, Benditt EP: Clustering of replicating cells in aortic endothelium. Proc Natl Acad Sci USA 73:651–654, 1976.

Skalak R, Nerem RM, editors: Biomechanics Symposium, Applied Mechanics Conference, at the Rensselaer Polytechnic Institute, Troy, N.Y. 1975.

Stamler J: Atherosclerotic coronary heart disease—Etiology and pathogenesis: The epidemiologic findings. Lectures on Preventive Cardiology, edited by J Stamler, pp. 63–78. New York: Grune & Stratton, 1967.

Stamler J: Epidemiology of coronary heart disease. Med Clin North Am 57:5–46, 1973.

Stamler J: Primary prevention of sudden coronary death. Circulation 52 (Suppl 3):III-258–III-279, 1975.

Stehbens WE: Intracranial arterial aneurysms and atherosclerosis. Thesis, University of Sydney, 1958.

Stehbens WE: Focal intimal proliferation in the cerebral arteries. Am J Pathol 36:289, 1960.

Stehbens WE: Flow in experimental models simulating intravascular cords traversing the arterial lumen. Vasc Surg 9:132–140, 1975.

Stehbens WE: The role of hemodynamics in the pathogenesis of atherosclerosis. Prog Cardiovasc Dis 18:89–103, 1975.

Talbot L. Berger SA: Fluid-mechanical aspects of the human circulation. Am Sci 62:671–682, 1974.

Texon M: The hemodynamic concept of atherosclerosis—A product of scientific integration. In: Medicine, Science and the Law, pp. 251–259. London: Sweet and Maxwell, Ltd, 1961.

Vital Statistics Reports (Supplement), Vol. 25 No. 11. National Center for Health Statistics, U.S. Dept of Health, Education, and Welfare, 1977.

Walker WJ: Changing United States life-style and declining vascular mortality: Cause or coincidence? N Engl J Med 297:163–165, 1977.

Yih GS: An Introduction to Fluid Mechanics. New York: McGraw-Hill, 1969.

Zalosh RG, Nelson WG: Pulsating flow in a curved tube. J Fluid Mechanics 59:693, 1973.

INDEX